Intravenous Infusion Therapy Skills Checklists

Intravenous Infusion Therapy Skills Checklists

Dianne L. Josephson, RN, MSN

Infusion Therapy Consultant, El Paso, Texas
Nursing Education Consultant Services, El Paso, Texas

THOMSON

DELMAR LEARNING

Australia   Canada   Mexico   Singapore   Spain   United Kingdom   United States

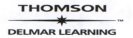

THOMSON

DELMAR LEARNING

Intravenous Infusion Therapy Skills Checklists
by Dianne L. Josephson

Vice President, Health Care Business Unit:
William Brottmiller

Director of Learning Solutions:
Matthew Kane

Acquisitions Editor:
Maureen Rosener

Senior Product Manager:
Elisabeth F. Williams

Marketing Director:
Jennifer McAvey

Marketing Channel Manager:
Michelle McTighe

Marketing Coordinator:
Danielle Pacella

Production Director:
Carolyn Miller

Production Editor:
Jack Pendleton

Library of Congress Cataloging-in-Publication Data

Josephson, Dianne L.
  Intravenous infusion therapy skills checklists / Dianne L. Josephson.
    p. cm.
  Includes bibliographical references and index.
  ISBN 1-4018-6499-6 (alk. paper)
  1. Infusion therapy. 2. Nursing. I. Title.
  RM170.J69 2006
  615.5—dc22

                                2006014987

NOTICE TO THE READER

Contents

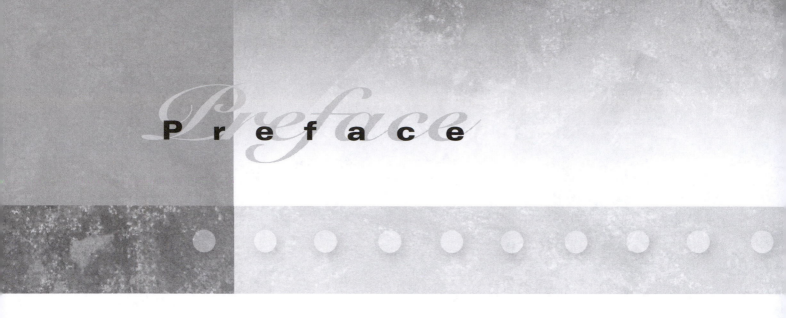

Preface

Intravenous infusion therapy is a key nursing responsibility. Practitioners are charged with safe patient care through preparation, setup, administration, and follow-up care related to IV administration of medication. Excellent technique, thorough knowledge, and precision in execution are all needed to ensure safe practice.

Intravenous Infusion Therapy Skills Checklists is a must-have reference for any professional who is performing procedures and wants to become a safe practitioner. Skills checklists will allow users to judge their competence in performing 37 different IV therapy procedures. Skills range from Preparing the Infusion Site to Starting an IV, to Flushing the CVC and Transfusion of Blood Components.

A consistent format is used to present each skill, starting with skill overview and time requirements. Step-by-step instructions on carrying out the procedure are detailed with all the information necessary for accurate technique. Space is allotted for evaluating success in completing the skill, and a column for notes encourages users to keep track of tips and thoughts for improving their technique. All these features combine to make each skill complete and user-friendly.

SPECIAL REVIEWER AND CONSULTANT

Rosemary Gangemi, RN, MSN

Memorial Hospital
Gulfport, Mississippi

and

Adjunct faculty
University of Southern Mississippi—Gulf Park
Long Beach, Mississippi

Skill 1 | Tourniquet Application

Name _____ Date _____ Instructor _____

Approximate Time to Complete the Skill: 2–3 minutes

Overview of the Skill

A tourniquet is a constrictive device used to temporarily impede blood flow (venous return) in an extremity that is distal to the site of its application. It is typically made from rubber tubing or a strip of Velcro®. A blood pressure cuff may serve as a tourniquet when it is inflated to a reading midway between a client's systolic and diastolic pressures or just below the diastolic pressure. The force created by the tourniquet serves to provide venous distension. A tourniquet is implemented to distend the vein prior to venipuncture so the vein is more readily palpable or visible, thereby alleviating unnecessary trauma during cannulation.

When using a tourniquet, the most important thing to keep in mind is to apply it so that it only suppresses venous—not arterial—blood flow. To ensure this, the nurse always must be able to palpate or auscultate a pulse distal to the tourniquet. Tissue damage can occur if arterial blood flow is impeded or if the tourniquet remains in place for an extended time. Tourniquets should be removed as soon as possible.

ACTION TAKEN	COMPLETED SUCCESSFULLY	DID NOT COMPLETE	NOTES
1. Check the physician's order.			
2. Introduce yourself to the patient.			
3. Identify the patient by checking the wristband against the doctor's order and asking the patient, if conscious, to state his/her name.			
4. Verify the patient's allergy status.			
5. Explain the proposed procedure in terms the patient can understand.			
6. Carry out proper hand hygiene.			
7. Gather equipment.			
8. Provide for the patient's privacy.			
9. To apply the tourniquet correctly, hold one end in the dominant hand and the other end in the nondominant hand.			

(continues)

Skill 1 | *(continued)*

Name _____ Date _____ Instructor _____

ACTION TAKEN	COMPLETED SUCCESSFULLY	DID NOT COMPLETE	NOTES
10. Encircle the extremity 3 to 4 inches above the venipuncture site and lay one length over the other, close to the skin, as if tying a knot. The end of the tubing in the nurse's dominant hand is not brought through completely (as it would be if tying a knot) but, rather, is tucked under the other segment.			
11. Assess for a pulse distal to the application site.			
12. To remove the tourniquet, pull the end of the tucked portion.			

Skill 2 | Primary Infusion Setup

Name _____ Date _____ Instructor _____

Approximate Time to Complete the Skill: 8 minutes

Overview of the Skill

Prior to starting an intravenous infusion, the correct infusate has to be set up with a primary administration set. If piggyback medications or secondary infusions are ordered or anticipated, the nurse should procure a set that has a back-check valve and injection ports. The interior of the tubing, both ends of the tubing, and the IV fluid all have to be kept sterile to avoid contamination. Gravity flow tubing, or tubing that is not pump-specific, is available in macrodrip (usually 15 drops per ml) and microdrip (usually 60 drops per ml).

There are many tubings specific for a variety of IV pumps. Although the principles for setting up the infusion remain the same, directions should be checked for any specific tubing, as manufacturer's instructions may have slight variations for setting up their particular brand of tubing.

ACTION TAKEN	COMPLETED SUCCESSFULLY	DID NOT COMPLETE	NOTES
1. Check the physician's order.			
2. Introduce yourself to the patient.			
3. Identify the patient by checking the wristband against the doctor's order and asking the patient, if conscious, to state his/her name.			
4. Verify the patient's allergy status.			
5. Explain the proposed procedure in terms the patient can understand.			
6. Carry out proper hand hygiene.			
7. Gather the ordered IV fluids, appropriate tubing, and a clean IV pole for setup in an uncontaminated area away from the patient's room. If a pole-mounted EID (electronic infusion device) is needed, check to be sure that it is in proper working order and that the batteries are charged.			

(continues)

Skill 2 | *(continued)*

Name _____ Date _____ Instructor _____

ACTION TAKEN	COMPLETED SUCCESSFULLY	DID NOT COMPLETE	NOTES
8. Check the IV fluid for type and amount, expiration date, clarity, and leaks in the bag or bottle. For plastic infusate containers, remove the outer tear-off wrap, following the manufacturer's directions. (This wrap will have been removed in the pharmacy if an admixture has been ordered.)			
9. Check the expiration date on the IV tubing container, then open it. Ensure that the sterile cover is over the infusate spike and that the distal end, where the IV cannula connects, is intact. (If the cannula end has a "breathable" attachment, it will not have a cover over it.) Once the set is removed from its package, keep it coiled and contained above waist level.			
10. Close the roller clamp on the administration set tubing (but not the slide clamps, if any).			
11. Hang the plastic bags containing the IV fluids on an IV pole.			
12. Place glass containers on a clean counter.			

Skill 2 | *(continued)*

Name _____ Date _____ Instructor _____

ACTION TAKEN	COMPLETED SUCCESSFULLY	DID NOT COMPLETE	NOTES
13a. To spike a plastic bag: (1) Secure the neck of the bag with the thumb and index finger of the nondominant hand and remove the sterile cover on the administration set port with the dominant hand. (2) Remove the sterile cover from the tubing administration set spike. Do not touch the spike itself. (3) Grasp the middle of the outside surface of the administration port, holding it vertically between the thumb and index and third fingers of the nondominant hand. Holding the finger-guard area below the spiked portion of the administration set, insert the spike into the administration port, using a straight, twisting motion.			
OR			
13b. To spike a glass bottle: (1) Be sure to use the appropriate administration set. A vented set must be used if the bottle has no internal venting system.			

(continues)

Skill 2 | *(continued)*

Name _____ Date _____ Instructor _____

ACTION TAKEN	COMPLETED SUCCESSFULLY	DID NOT COMPLETE	NOTES
(2) With the bottle standing upright on a level surface, hold it in place with the non-dominant hand and, with the dominant hand, peel off the outer aluminum band from the top of the bottle.			
(3) Remove the rubber disk stopper, which seals the vacuum and sterile lid of the bottle where the administration port sits. If an admixture has been instilled, the aluminum cap and rubber stopper will have been removed in the pharmacy and sealed with a tamperproof closure, which must be torn off before spiking. Do not touch the top of the bottle where the administration port or vent outlet sits. If it is touched, wipe the top thoroughly with a 70% alcohol solution prior to spiking.			
(4) Remove the sterile cap from the spike and push it into the port with a straight (not twisting) movement.			

Skill 2 | *(continued)*

Name _____ Date _____ Instructor _____

ACTION TAKEN	COMPLETED SUCCESSFULLY	DID NOT COMPLETE	NOTES
(5) Suspend the bottle on the IV pole by the aluminum bale at the bottom of the container.			
14. Squeeze the drip chamber to allow it to fill one-third to one-half full or to the level of the manufacturer's imprinted marking on the chamber.			
15. Remove the sterile cap from the distal end of the administration set. Be sure to maintain the sterility of the cap. Prime the administration tubing by holding the distal end of the administration set over (but not touching) a basin, paper towel, or sink. Slowly open the roller clamp to purge air from the set. As the fluid approaches the check valve or any injection ports, invert those sites and tap on them to remove any trapped air.			
16. Once the infusate reaches the distal end of the administration set and there are no visible air pockets, clamp the tubing or recap it (as appropriate), and hang it over the top of the IV pole for transport to the patient's room.			

(continues)

Name _____ Date _____ Instructor _____

ACTION TAKEN	COMPLETED SUCCESSFULLY	DID NOT COMPLETE	NOTES
17. Add connectors and add-on devices before or after priming, depending on the manufacturer's guidelines. The priming volume is stated on the packaging.			
18. Label the infusate container and the administration set with the date and the time, per institutional policy.			
19. Adjust the height of the infusate container to approximately 36 inches above the intended IV insertion site.			

Skill 3 | Preparing the Infusion Site

Name _____ Date _____ Instructor _____

Approximate Time to Complete the Skill: 5 minutes

Overview of the Skill

Preparing the infusion site properly is necessary to prevent injury and to avoid introducing microorganisms that could predispose an individual to infection. The skin can be prepared using 2% aqueous chlorhexidine gluconate, 70% isopropyl alcohol, and povidone-iodine or 70% tincture of iodine.

When the intended area of venipuncture has hair sufficient to impede venous visualization, site disinfection, cannula insertion, or adherence to the dressing, the hair can be removed by gently clipping with scissors close to the skin without scratching the epidermis. Because of the potential for microabrasion and the introduction of contaminants, the hair should not be shaved. Nor should depilatories be applied for hair removal because of the possibility of irritating the skin or inciting allergic reactions. Depending on agency policy, an electric shaver may be used, if it belongs to the patient or if the shaving heads can be changed or disinfected between use with different patients.

ACTION TAKEN	COMPLETED SUCCESSFULLY	DID NOT COMPLETE	NOTES
1. Check the physician's order.			
2. Introduce yourself to the patient.			
3. Identify the patient by checking the wristband against the doctor's order and asking the patient, if conscious, to state his/her name.			
4. Verify the patient's allergy status.			
5. Explain the proposed procedure in terms the patient can understand.			
6. Carry out proper hand hygiene.			
7. Gather all necessary equipment.			
8. Choose the most appropriate vein.			
9. Assess for intact, unbruised skin.			
10. If excessive hair is present, clip short with scissors.			

(continues)

Skill 3 | *(continued)*

Name _____ Date _____ Instructor _____

ACTION TAKEN	COMPLETED SUCCESSFULLY	DID NOT COMPLETE	NOTES
11. Using friction, cleanse the site with 70% isopropyl alcohol, beginning at the intended cannulation site and working outward 2 to 3 inches, in a concentric circle, for 20 to 30 seconds. Do not backtrack over a previously cleaned area. Allow the alcohol to air-dry. Do not blow on or fan the skin, and do not wipe the alcohol off the area.			
12. Using the same directional movement, cleanse the site thoroughly with 2% aqueous chlorhexidine gluconate, povidone-iodine, or tincture of iodine. If tincture of iodine is used, wipe the site gently with a sterile gauze.			
13. Proceed with venipuncture.			

Skill 4 | Starting an IV: Over-the-Needle Catheter

Name _____ Date _____ Instructor _____

Approximate Time to Complete the Skill: 15 minutes

Overview of the Skill

The most commonly used angiocatheter to start an infusion is the over-the-needle catheter (ONC). An ONC is a flexible catheter, encased in a metal stylet that is used to pierce the skin and vein and attaches to the infusion tubing (after the stylet has been removed). The ONC has essentially replaced straight steel needles that once were the main device to deliver fluids into the vein.

ACTION TAKEN	COMPLETED SUCCESSFULLY	DID NOT COMPLETE	NOTES
1. Check the physician's order.			
2. Introduce yourself to the patient.			
3. Identify the patient by checking the wristband against the doctor's order and asking the patient, if conscious, to state his/her name.			
4. Verify the patient's allergy status.			
5. Explain the proposed procedure in terms the patient can understand.			
6. Carry out proper hand hygiene.			
7. Set up all the necessary supplies on the bedside stand or overbed table in the order in which they will be used.			
8. Cut any tape that will be needed.			
9. Inspect the ONC to be sure the needle bevel is sharp and smooth, and read the manufacturer's directions regarding inspection and manipulation of the ONC.			
10. Provide privacy to the patient and elevate the bed level.			

(continues)

Skill 4 | *(continued)*

Name _____ Date _____ Instructor _____

ACTION TAKEN	COMPLETED SUCCESSFULLY	DID NOT COMPLETE	NOTES
11. Place the patient in a Fowler's or semi-Fowler's position with the extremity intended for cannulation below the level of the patient's heart.			
12. Protect the patient's clothing and bedding with underpad or towel.			
13. Apply the tourniquet (see Skill 1), and identify the most appropriate vein for cannulation, preferably in the patient's nondominant hand. a. Select a vein, using the most distal vein first. b. Avoid bony prominences. c. Avoid areas of rash or broken skin.			
14. Remove the tourniquet and leave it under the extremity.			
15. If the venipuncture site has excessive hair, clip the hair at the site. Do not shave the area.			
16. Antiseptically prepare the site according to policy.			
17. Don gloves.			
18. Apply tourniquet to occlude venous flow.			
19. Palpate for and ensure the presence of a pulse distal to the tourniquet.			

Skill 4 | *(continued)*

Name _____ Date _____ Instructor _____

ACTION TAKEN	COMPLETED SUCCESSFULLY	DID NOT COMPLETE	NOTES
20. Remove the needle cover and instruct the patient that the needle will be entering the vein.			
21. With gentle skin traction, anchor the vein below the intended insertion site and, using the thumb of your non-dominant hand, pull the skin taut.			
22. Hold the ONC by the needle hub flash chamber (not the color-coded hub of the catheter unit), with the bevel up.			
23. Enter the over-the-needle catheter via either a direct method or an indirect method. a. *Direct-entry method:* Position the needle over the vein with the needle in the bevel-up position and pointing in the direction of the blood flow. In this method, the needle passes through the skin, over and directly into the vein in one maneuver. b. *Indirect-entry method:* Position the needle in the bevel-up position and alongside the vein, pointing in the direction of the blood flow. In this method, the needle enters the skin, is maneuvered alongside the vein, and then enters the vein.			

(continues)

Skill 4 | *(continued)*

Name _____ Date _____ Instructor _____

ACTION TAKEN	COMPLETED SUCCESSFULLY	DID NOT COMPLETE	NOTES
24. Hold the needle at a 15-degree angle for insertion into superficial veins and a 25- to 30-degree angle for insertion into deeper veins.			
25. Observe for flash-back of blood in the flash chamber. *Note:* Upon entry into the tunica adventitia (outermost) layer of the vein, the nurse may feel a slight "pop" (or sensation of release of pressure), depending on the brand of catheter used. Some of the newer types, such as those made with Vialon®, provide such a sharp, smooth insertion that there is little or no characteristic "pop" upon vein access.			
26. Once the over-the-needle catheter is in the vein, lower the needle until it is almost flush with the skin to avoid puncturing the opposite wall of the vein, then advance the needle and catheter unit so the tip of the catheter is in the center of the vein lumen.			
27. Advance the catheter, using one of the following techniques: • Advance the whole unit—needle and catheter—into the vein, then retract the needle.			

Skill 4 | *(continued)*

Name _____ Date _____ Instructor _____

ACTION TAKEN	COMPLETED SUCCESSFULLY	DID NOT COMPLETE	NOTES
• Stabilize the needle flash chamber, and gradually advance the catheter off the needle, threading it into the vein lumen until the desired length has been inserted. If the catheter does not thread smoothly or blood flow ceases, remove the catheter and needle together, apply pressure to the site, and attempt venipuncture in another site, using a new device. • *In the hooding method:* Hold the catheter unit stationary and advance the catheter off the needle no more than 1/4 inch, hooding the tip of the needle inside the catheter. If preferred, pull the needle back no more than 1/4 inch to achieve the same result. Grasp the color-coded catheter hub and advance the hooded needle or catheter as a unit into the vein. When it is in place, remove the needle.			

(continues)

Skill 4 | *(continued)*

Name _____ Date _____ Instructor _____

ACTION TAKEN	COMPLETED SUCCESSFULLY	DID NOT COMPLETE	NOTES
• *In the floating method:* Advance the needle and catheter about halfway into the vein (verified by flashback), at which point remove the tourniquet and needle. Then attach the cannula hub to the infusion tubing, slowly open the flow control clamp, and start the infusion. Then float the catheter into the vein with the infusate. *Note:* For this method to work well, the skin and vein must remain anchored with one hand. If anchoring is not maintained, the catheter may meet resistance from skin traction at the insertion site.			
28. Release the tourniquet without touching the end of the catheter hub or the IV insertion site. If desired, place a sterile 2 × 2-inch gauze pad under the catheter hub.			
29. Remove the needle and dispose of it in the sharps container.			
30. Connect the infusion tubing with a gentle push-and-twist motion.			
31. Place a strip of paper tape over the tubing.			

Skill 4 | *(continued)*

Name _____ Date _____ Instructor _____

ACTION TAKEN	COMPLETED SUCCESSFULLY	DID NOT COMPLETE	NOTES
32. Open the flow clamp and observe the insertion site and vessel pathway as the infusate freely enters the vessel. Adjust the flow rate.			
33. Remove the strip of paper tape and dress the site per agency policy.			
34. Remove gloves and carry out proper hand hygiene.			
35. Label the site at the side of the dressing with the date, time, IV device used, and your initials.			
36. Label the infusion container and all administration sets that are used.			
37. Return the bed to the lowest position, lower the head of the bed (if appropriate for the patient), and raise the bedrails.			

Skill 5 | Starting an IV: Winged Infusion Set

Name _____ Date _____ Instructor _____

Approximate Time to Complete the Skill: 15 minutes

Overview of the Skill

IV therapy can be administered through a winged infusion set, also known as a butterfly needle. This is a short metal needle that lies within the vein during infusion therapy. The needle extends from soft plastic wings and is connected to a short, permanently attached extension tubing. The wings provide a means to stabilize the cannula when secured with tape. The wings are flexible and can be bent upward to act as a handle when the needle is inserted.

Because this is a metal needle, there is an increased chance of the needle becoming dislodged during therapy. Winged steel needles usually are used to provide IV therapy to infants or for very short-term drug or fluid administration, such as a one-time order. Their use is generally a nursing judgment, based on accurate assessment, as to which type of device is most appropriate for a specific patient. The most common sites for inserting a winged needle are the dorsal surface of the hand and the smaller veins in the forearm.

ACTION TAKEN	COMPLETED SUCCESSFULLY	DID NOT COMPLETE	NOTES
1. Check the physician's order.			
2. Introduce yourself to the patient.			
3. Identify the patient by checking the wristband against the doctor's order and asking the patient, if conscious, to state his/her name.			
4. Verify the patient's allergy status.			
5. Explain the proposed procedure in terms the patient can understand.			
6. Carry out proper hand hygiene.			
7. Gather all necessary equipment.			
8. Provide for the patient's privacy.			
9. Assess for an appropriate vein in the patient's non-dominant hand/arm. A vein should be chosen at the most distal site, working upward in a proximal direction.			
10. Apply the tourniquet; for most patients this should be 2 to 3 inches above the intended venipuncture site.			

Skill 5 | *(continued)*

Name _____ Date _____ Instructor _____

ACTION TAKEN	COMPLETED SUCCESSFULLY	DID NOT COMPLETE	NOTES
11. Cleanse the skin with alcohol-prepped pad (or per agency policy) starting at the insertion site and working outward in a circular motion. Once the site is cleansed, do not retouch the site, unless with a sterile gloved finger or a gloved finger that has been prepped with 70% isopropyl alcohol.			
12. If the patient is not allergic, cleanse the skin with 2% aqueous chlorhexidine gluconate, povidone-iodine, or agency-approved iodophor (or per agency policy).			
13. While the iodophor is drying, don gloves.			
The following method works well for patients who have well-developed, elastic veins, with good venous pressure. 14. Hold taut the skin below the insertion site.			
15. Pick up the winged needle, holding it by the plastic wings, bevel up.			
16. Insert the needle with the bevel up at a 20- to 30-degree angle.			
17. Assess for retrograde blood flow into the tubing of the set.			
18. Apply a strip of paper tape across the wings.			

(continues)

Skill 5 | *(continued)*

Name _____ Date _____ Instructor _____

ACTION TAKEN	COMPLETED SUCCESSFULLY	DID NOT COMPLETE	NOTES
19. Allow retrograde blood flow to purge the tubing of air, then connect the medication syringe and administration set tubing for the infusion, or apply a male-adapter plug as appropriate and instill a saline lock.			
20. Apply the appropriate dressing.			
21. Remove the tourniquet.			
22. Write (to the side of the dressing or on a piece of tape or labeling) the date, time, needle size (length and gauge), and your initials.			
23. Make the patient comfortable.			
24. Document the procedure in the medical record in the nurse's notes and appropriate infusion flow sheets. If medications are administered, document in the Medication Administration Record (MAR).			
A variation in technique can be used when it is anticipated that backflow of blood into the winged set tubing will be sluggish, as follows: • Attach a syringe containing 3 to 5 ml of normal saline to the winged infusion set, and prime the tubing and the needle.			

Skill 6 | Adding Medication to an Infusion Container

Name _____ Date _____ Instructor _____

Approximate Time to Complete the Skill: 8 minutes

Overview of the Skill

In general, admixtures are dispensed directly into infusate containers in the pharmacy. Admixing is done under laminar air-flow hoods. Laminar air-flow refers to air that moves along separate but parallel flow paths into filters where contaminants are removed.

In the not-too-distant past, nurses commonly prepared their own admixtures for primary infusions. This is no longer considered safe practice, so nurses should not carry out that procedure.

ACTION TAKEN	COMPLETED SUCCESSFULLY	DID NOT COMPLETE	NOTES
1. Check the physician's order.			
2. Introduce yourself to the patient.			
3. Identify the patient by checking the wristband against the doctor's order and asking the patient, if conscious, to state his/her name.			
4. Verify the patient's allergy status.			
5. Explain the proposed procedure in terms the patient can understand.			
6. Carry out proper hand hygiene.			
7. Gather necessary equipment.			
8. Check the medication for the name, dosage, expiration date, appropriate appearance, and integrity of the container.			
9. Draw up the medication dose as prescribed.			
10. Clamp the tubing on the infusate administration tubing.			
11. Remove the infusion container from the IV pole.			

(continues)

Skill 6 | *(continued)*

Name _____ Date _____ Instructor _____

ACTION TAKEN	COMPLETED SUCCESSFULLY	DID NOT COMPLETE	NOTES
12. Swab the injection port on the infusate container with alcohol.			
13. Inject the medication into the injection port.			
14. Gently rock the infusion container back and forth.			
15. Hang the container on the IV pole.			
16. Discard the used syringe into the sharps container.			
17. Open the clamp on the IV tubing and regulate the rate of flow.			
18. Stay with the patient for five minutes.			
19. Affix a label to the infusate container to indicate the addition of the drug. The label should contain: a. name of drug b. dose of drug c. date d. time the drug was added e. amount of infusate in container when drug was added f. expiration time g. nurse's name.			
20. Carry out proper hand hygiene.			
21. Document in the Medication Administration Record (MAR).			

Skill 7 | IV Piggyback

Name _____ Date _____ Instructor _____

Approximate Time to Complete the Skill: 5 minutes

Overview of the Skill

A secondary infusion is initiated after the primary infusion is already in progress. This is the most common method to administer IV medications concurrently with the primary infusion. The ordered medication is diluted in a small volume IV container (usually 50–100 ml) of compatible infusate. The secondary line (piggyback) is coupled to the primary line at the first injection port below the back-check valve.

The piggyback can function concurrently with a primary infusion only when it is suspended higher than the primary line (which must have a back-check valve). By opening the clamp on the secondary line, the primary infusion temporarily stops flowing. When the piggyback infusion is complete and the infusate in its tubing falls below the level of the primary line drip chamber, the back-check valve opens and the primary infusion resumes.

ACTION TAKEN	COMPLETED SUCCESSFULLY	DID NOT COMPLETE	NOTES
1. Check the physician's order.			
2. Introduce yourself to the patient.			
3. Identify the patient by checking the wristband against the doctor's order and asking the patient, if conscious, to state his/her name.			
4. Verify the patient's allergy status.			
5. Explain the proposed procedure in terms the patient can understand.			
6. Carry out proper hand hygiene.			
7. Provide privacy to the patient.			

(continues)

Skill 7 | *(continued)*

Name _____ Date _____ Instructor _____

ACTION TAKEN	COMPLETED SUCCESSFULLY	DID NOT COMPLETE	NOTES
8. Obtain the medication, verify that it is correct and compatible with the current infusate, and check the expiration date. If the medication is refrigerated, it should be removed from the refriger-ator 20 to 30 minutes before administration. If the medication is stored at room temperature, it should be opened immediately before administration.			
9. Set up all the necessary supplies, and don gloves.			
10. Open the sterile container with the secondary medica-tion administration set.			
11. Clamp the sec-ondary medication administration set and spike the med-ication container without contami-nating it.			
12. Do not fill the drip chamber, and do not prime the tubing in the con-ventional manner.			
13. Use alcohol to swab the injection port directly below the check valve on the primary tubing.			
14. Attach the secondary tubing to the cleansed injection port with the appropriate needle or needle-less adapter.			

Skill 7 | *(continued)*

Name _____ Date _____ Instructor _____

ACTION TAKEN	COMPLETED SUCCESSFULLY	DID NOT COMPLETE	NOTES
15. While the primary infusate is still running, lower the secondary bag below the level of the port into which it is tethered.			
16. Slowly open the clamp on the secondary administration set and let the infusate from the primary line purge the secondary tubing of air (via retrograde fluid flow). When the drip chamber is one-half to two-thirds full, close the roller clamp on the secondary set.			
17. Attach the hanger, included in the secondary set, to the primary infusate container (making the primary container hang lower than the secondary container).			
18. Open the roller clamp on the secondary tubing and infuse the piggybacked infusate at the prescribed rate. Do not close the clamp on the primary infusion.			
19. Tape or affix a manufactured coupling device to secure the connection between the primary and secondary lines.			
20. Assess the patient's response.			
21. Document in the Medication Administration Record (MAR).			

Skill 8 | IV Drug Administration into an Existing Infusion Line

Name _____ Date _____ Instructor _____

Approximate Time to Complete the Skill: 5 minutes

Overview of the Skill

Intravenous medications can be administered into an existing infusion line. In this form of administering medication, the primary infusate is stopped for a short time while an intravenous medication is instilled into the primary tubing via an injection port close to the patient. Once the medication is administered, the primary infusion is resumed. The nurse must perform any required nursing interventions that accompany administration of medication, including checking vital signs and informing patients of the purpose and sensations or side effects of the medication.

Two important considerations while administering a medication in this manner are (1) recognizing compatibility or incompatibility between the medication to be injected and the existing infusate, and (2) delivering the medication at the appropriate rate. If the medication and infusate are not compatible, saline is used to flush the tubing both before and after administering the medicine. Rate of administration of the medication is determined by the amount of medicine to be given in one minute. Before administering the medication, the nurse should verify the rate of administration by checking with the physician's order, the physician, the pharmacist, or a drug reference book.

ACTION TAKEN	COMPLETED SUCCESSFULLY	DID NOT COMPLETE	NOTES
1. Check the physician's order, and verify the rate of administration.			
2. Introduce yourself to the patient.			
3. Identify the patient by checking the wristband against the doctor's order and asking the patient, if conscious, to state his/her name.			
4. Verify the patient's allergy status.			
5. Explain the proposed procedure in terms the patient can understand.			
6. Carry out proper hand hygiene.			
7. Provide privacy to the patient.			
8. Elevate the bed level.			
9. Assess vital signs and level of consciousness, and record.			
10. Set up necessary supplies on the bedside stand or overbed table in the order in which they will be used.			

Skill 8 | *(continued)*

Name _____ Date _____ Instructor _____

ACTION TAKEN	COMPLETED SUCCESSFULLY	DID NOT COMPLETE	NOTES
11. Ascertain that the medication to be injected is compatible with the existing infusion. (If it is not compatible, the injection must be preceded and followed by normal saline [or manufacturer-provided diluent] while the infusate flow in the tubing above the injection site is stopped, either by pinching off or using the slide clamp on the tubing set.)			
12. Don gloves.			
13. Swab the injection port nearest to the patient with alcohol.			
14. Insert needle or needless adapter into the port.			
15. Stop the primary infusion by pinching shut the administration set tubing just behind the injection port (or, if the administration set has a slide clamp, close it).			
16. Inject the medication according to directions.			
17. Remove the syringe or needle and dispose of it properly in the sharps container.			
18. Check to be sure the infusion is running at the appropriate rate, and adjust as required to maintain the schedule.			
19. Return bed to normal position.			

Skill 9 | Using a Peripheral Intermittent Infusion Device

Name _____ Date _____ Instructor _____

Approximate Time to Complete the Skill: 5 minutes

Overview of the Skill

An intermittent infusion device or plug (saline lock), also called a male adapter plug (and formerly called a heparin lock), is used to keep an IV line available once a primary infusion is no longer needed. It consists of a small, resealable apparatus or cap that accommodates a needle or needleless access device that is screwed, via a Luer-Lok™ connector, onto the hub of an IV cannula. It may be used to administer intermittent medications. It can be reattached to IV tubing if infusion therapy is needed again.

ACTION TAKEN	COMPLETED SUCCESSFULLY	DID NOT COMPLETE	NOTES
1. Check the physician's order.			
2. Introduce yourself to the patient.			
3. Identify the patient by checking the wristband against the doctor's order and asking the patient, if conscious, to state his/her name.			
4. Verify the patient's allergy status.			
5. Explain the proposed procedure in terms the patient can understand.			
6. Carry out proper hand hygiene.			
7. Provide privacy to the patient.			
8. Elevate the bed level.			
9. Set up necessary supplies on the bedside stand or overbed table in the order they will be used.			
10. Don gloves.			
11. Open the sterile container with the intermittent injection plug, remove the sterile cap, attach the syringe of normal saline, prime the plug, and leave the syringe attached.			

Skill 9 | *(continued)*

Name _____ Date _____ Instructor _____

ACTION TAKEN	COMPLETED SUCCESSFULLY	DID NOT COMPLETE	NOTES
12. Stop the infusion.			
13. Loosen the existing infusion tubing, remove the tubing, remove the sterile cap (if present) on the Luer-Lok®, and insert the intermittent infusion plug. Screw it securely onto the cannula hub.			
14. Open the slide clamp on the set, aspirate, and slowly inject the saline. Stop injecting when the last 0.5 ml of saline remains, and immediately close the slide clamp on the set.			
15. Dispose of the syringe in the sharps container.			
16. Properly dispose of the infusate and tubing.			
17. Remove gloves and carry out proper hand hygiene.			
18. Document in the nurse's notes assessment data regarding the site, discontinuation of the primary infusion, and evaluation of the patient's response to the procedure.			

Skill 10 | Discontinuation of an IV

Name _____ Date _____ Instructor _____

Approximate Time to Complete the Skill: 7 minutes

Overview of the Skill

A peripheral infusion line is discontinued when it is no longer needed. It may be terminated by order of the physician or when complications dictate that it is to be stopped.

ACTION TAKEN	COMPLETED SUCCESSFULLY	DID NOT COMPLETE	NOTES
1. Check the physician's order.			
2. Introduce yourself to the patient.			
3. Identify the patient by checking the wristband against the doctor's order and asking the patient, if conscious, to state his/her name.			
4. Verify the patient's allergy status.			
5. Explain the proposed procedure in terms the patient can understand.			
6. Carry out proper hand hygiene.			
7. Gather necessary supplies.			
8. Provide privacy to the patient.			
9. Elevate the bed.			
10. Clamp infusion tubing and turn off electronic infusion device (if appropriate).			
11. Cut or tear off a few strips of tape.			
12. Don gloves.			

Skill 10 | *(continued)*

Name _____ Date _____ Instructor _____

ACTION TAKEN	COMPLETED SUCCESSFULLY	DID NOT COMPLETE	NOTES
13. Remove all tape and carefully loosen the skin from the edges of the dressing over the IV site, using the stretch method or alcohol (or adhesive remover) method. Be careful not to pull on the cannula.			
14. While stabilizing the cannula hub, remove the entire IV dressing, moving in the direction of the IV device, not away from it.			
15. Place a 2 × 2-inch sterile gauze (not alcohol) over the IV insertion site, and apply gentle pressure while grasping the cannula hub and removing the catheter with one smooth movement.			
16. Place the catheter on the paper towel.			
17. Elevate the extremity and apply firm, gentle pressure to the IV site for 60 seconds, or until there is no bleeding.			
18. Assess the site and apply tape firmly over the gauze. If the patient is undergoing anticoagulation therapy or has a bleeding disorder, a larger pressure dressing may be needed.			
19. Examine the removed catheter.			

(continues)

Skill 10 | *(continued)*

Name _____ Date _____ Instructor _____

ACTION TAKEN	COMPLETED SUCCESSFULLY	DID NOT COMPLETE	NOTES
20. Dispose of the IV device in the sharps container.			
21. Return the bed to the lowest position and raise the bedrails.			
22. Recheck the IV site.			
23. Document in the nurse's notes assessment data regarding the site and removed catheter, discontinuation of the infusion, and evaluation of the patient's response to the procedure.			

Skill 11 | Medication Administration by Bolus Delivery

Name _____ Date _____ Instructor _____

Approximate Time to Complete the Skill: 15–20 minutes

Overview of the Skill

When an intravenous medication is administered to a patient without established intravenous access, a needle and syringe may be used. If a patient is to receive more than one dose of medication over a period of time, a saline lock or other intravenous device should be ordered and initiated.

ACTION TAKEN	COMPLETED SUCCESSFULLY	DID NOT COMPLETE	NOTES
1. Check the physician's order.			
2. Introduce yourself to the patient.			
3. Identify the patient by checking the wristband against the doctor's order and asking the patient, if conscious, to state his/her name.			
4. Verify the patient's allergy status.			
5. Explain the proposed procedure in terms the patient can understand.			
6. Carry out proper hand hygiene.			
7. Draw up the medication in a syringe.			
8. Change the needle, attaching the smallest one that will deliver the ordered medication and still accommodate the patient's vein.			
9. Perform any preadministration nursing interventions, such as taking vital signs or performing neurologic or cardiovascular assessments.			

(continues)

Skill 11 | *(continued)*

Name _____ Date _____ Instructor _____

ACTION TAKEN	COMPLETED SUCCESSFULLY	DID NOT COMPLETE	NOTES
10. Cut or tear one 4-inch strip of tape and open the 2 × 2-inch gauze without contaminating it.			
11. Apply the tourniquet and engorge the vein.			
12. Prep the site, using appropriate antiseptics. Work in a circular motion from the intended venipuncture site outward, extending to 2 inches. Do not backtrack. Allow the site to dry.			
13. Don gloves.			
14. Access the vein and pull back on the plunger to verify placement in the vein.			
15. Remove the tourniquet.			
16. Inject the medication.			
17. Place the 2 × 2-inch gauze over the injection site and remove the needle.			
18. Elevate the extremity until bleeding stops, and apply tape over the gauze.			
19. Dispose of the syringe properly in the sharps container to prevent needlestick injury and adhere to safety guidelines.			
20. Remove gloves and carry out proper hand hygiene.			

Skill 11 | *(continued)*

Name _____ Date _____ Instructor _____

ACTION TAKEN	COMPLETED SUCCESSFULLY	DID NOT COMPLETE	NOTES
21. Stay with the patient and assess his/her response to the medication.			
22. Perform any postadministration nursing interventions associated with the medication.			

Skill 12 | Medication Administration by Bolus Delivery Using a Winged-Administration Set

Name _____ Date _____ Instructor _____

Approximate Time to Complete the Skill: 15–20 minutes

Overview of Skill

A winged-administration set can be used to administer IV medication when an existing IV line is not in place and administration will take longer than a minute. The winged-administration set allows the nurse to assume a more comfortable position during administration of medication, since the wings help stabilize the needle. Care still must be taken to prevent dislodgement because this is a steel needle. If a patient is to receive more than one dose of medication over a period of time, a saline lock or other intravenous device should be ordered and initiated.

ACTION TAKEN	COMPLETED SUCCESSFULLY	DID NOT COMPLETE	NOTES
1. Check the physician's order.			
2. Introduce yourself to the patient.			
3. Identify the patient by checking the wristband against the doctor's order and asking the patient, if conscious, to state his/her name.			
4. Verify the patient's allergy status.			
5. Explain the proposed procedure in terms the patient can understand.			
6. Carry out proper hand hygiene.			
7. Draw up the medication into a syringe, and cap the needle.			
8. Draw up 2 to 3 ml of normal saline (0.9%) in each of two separate syringes and cap the needles.			
9. Attach a winged-administration set, with the smallest needle that will deliver the drug and be appropriate for the patient's vein, to one of the syringes containing 0.9% saline, and prime the tubing and needle on the set.			

Skill 12 | *(continued)*

Name _____ Date _____ Instructor _____

ACTION TAKEN	COMPLETED SUCCESSFULLY	DID NOT COMPLETE	NOTES
10. Perform any preadministration nursing interventions, such as taking vital signs or performing neurologic or cardiovascular assessments.			
11. Cut or tear two 4-inch strips of tape, and open the sterile 2 × 2-inch gauze without contaminating it.			
12. Apply the tourniquet to restrict venous blood flow and engorge the vein to facilitate venous access.			
13. Prep the site using a circular motion extending 2 inches outward from the intended venipuncture site. Do not backtrack. Allow the site to dry.			
14. Don gloves.			
15. Remove the tourniquet to reestablish venous blood flow and facilitate IV delivery of medication.			
16. Using the syringe attached to the 0.9% saline, insert the winged needle. Verify placement by retracting the plunger. If it's in the vein, flatten the administration set wings and place a strip of tape over them, securing the set to the patient's extremity. Slowly inject the 0.9% saline.			

(continues)

Skill 12 | *(continued)*

Name _____ Date _____ Instructor _____

ACTION TAKEN	COMPLETED SUCCESSFULLY	DID NOT COMPLETE	NOTES
17. Disconnect the empty syringe and attach the syringe containing the medication to the administration tubing.			
18. Inject the medication within the prescribed time.			
19. When the medication has been administered, disconnect the empty syringe and attach the second syringe of 0.9% saline to the administration set tubing. Inject the normal saline.			
20. Remove the strip of tape, place the 2 × 2-inch gauze on the injection site, and remove the needle.			
21. Elevate the extremity and apply pressure to the injection site until bleeding stops. Apply the clean strip of tape over the gauze.			
22. Dispose of the syringes and the winged-administration set properly in the sharps container to prevent needlestick injury and adhere to safety guidelines.			
23. Remove gloves and carry out proper hand hygiene to prevent spread of infection.			
24. Stay with the patient and assess his/her response to the medication.			
25. Perform any postadministration nursing interventions.			

Skill 13 | CVC Dressing Change and Site Care

Name _____ Date _____ Instructor _____

Approximate Time to Complete the Skill: 10 minutes

Overview of the Skill

The central venous catheter (CVC) site provides a direct-entry route to the systemic circulation. Extreme care must be taken to keep the site clean and free from microbial growth. This is accomplished by meticulous inspection, care of the site, and dressing changes. The dressing application and change to a CVC entry site is to be performed only by nurses who are specially trained and authorized by the agency.

The Centers for Disease Control and Prevention recommends that a CVC site dressing be changed when it becomes damp, loose, or soiled, or when inspection of the catheter site or catheter change is necessary. The nurse is expected to follow agency policies and protocols regarding care and maintenance of the catheter site.

ACTION TAKEN	COMPLETED SUCCESSFULLY	DID NOT COMPLETE	NOTES
1. Check the physician's order.			
2. Introduce yourself to the patient.			
3. Identify the patient by checking the wristband against the doctor's order and asking the patient, if conscious, to state his/her name.			
4. Verify the patient's allergy status.			
5. Explain the proposed procedure in terms the patient can understand.			
6. Carry out proper hand hygiene.			
7. Provide for the patient's privacy.			
8. Elevate the bed level.			
9. Secure all necessary supplies.			
10. Carry out proper hand hygiene.			
11. Nurse and patient don masks.			
12. Don clean, disposable gloves.			

(continues)

Skill 13 | *(continued)*

Name _____ Date _____ Instructor _____

ACTION TAKEN	COMPLETED SUCCESSFULLY	DID NOT COMPLETE	NOTES
13. Gently remove the soiled dressing, maneuvering the skin from the dressing in the direction of (toward) the catheter insertion site rather than from the insertion site outward. If a transparent, semi-permeable membrane dressing, use the stretch method. Do not touch the catheter insertion site.			
14. Examine the dressing for purulent drainage or foul odor.			
15. Remove disposable gloves and carry out proper hand hygiene.			
16. Examine the catheter site for abnormalities, such as: a. catheter malposition or slippage b. erythema c. dilated vessels d. drainage (notify physician and obtain specimen for culture and sensitivity [C & S], per agency policy) e. induration f. loose or absent sutures (notify physician or appropriate personnel regarding resuturing, or obtain Steri-Strips®, per agency policy.) g. tenderness.			

Skill 13 | *(continued)*

Name _____ Date _____ Instructor _____

ACTION TAKEN	COMPLETED SUCCESSFULLY	DID NOT COMPLETE	NOTES
17. Remove outer plastic wrap from the kit and tape it to the bedside.			
18. Aseptically open the supplies.			
19. Don sterile gloves.			
20. Clean the CVC site slowly, using friction and moving from the insertion site outward (including the catheter and catheter junction hub) in a concentric circle, to include the full area that the final dressing will cover. The sequence for cleaning is as follows: a. Clean first with the alcohol swabsticks, removing all debris. Use each side of each swab, and use all three swabsticks. Do not use organic solvents such as acetone or ether. b. Allow the alcohol to dry completely. c. Clean with 2% aqueous chlorhexidine gluconate or the iodophor, using all that are in the dressing kit. Use each side of the swabstick.			

(continues)

Skill 13 | *(continued)*

Name _____ Date _____ Instructor _____

ACTION TAKEN	COMPLETED SUCCESSFULLY	DID NOT COMPLETE	NOTES
21. Apply an agency-approved dressing. If it is a transparent, semipermeable membrane (TSM) dressing, be sure it molds around the catheter and junction of the hub (and do not stretch it during application).			
22. Remove the gloves and discard, along with all used materials.			
23. Secure the CVC pigtails to the skin above the dressing site.			
24. To the side of the dressing, place the label with the date, time, and nurse's initials.			
25. Carry out proper hand hygiene.			
26. Document in the nurse's notes all assessment data regarding the site and condition of the removed dressing, appropriate intervention data, and evaluation of the patient's response to the procedure.			

Skill 14 | Flushing the CVC

Name _____ Date _____ Instructor _____

Approximate Time to Complete the Skill: 5 minutes

Overview of the Skill

Routine flushing or irrigating is one of the most important mechanisms used to maintain the patency of a central line and prevent occlusion. Occlusion of a central venous catheter (CVC) can occur for a variety of reasons, including:

- improper flushing or irrigation (failure to use pulsatile, push-pause flushing)
- clot formation at lumen exit
- obstruction by drug precipitates
- obstruction by lipid deposition
- catheter displacement
- restriction of catheter flow by sutures that have tightened around the circumference of the catheter
- coiling, kinking, or pinching of the catheter between the clavicle and the first rib
- catheter damage or transection from repeated pressure of clavicle and first rib on the catheter during normal movement if it is placed through the "pinch-off" area.

Central lines should be flushed after every infusion, whenever the line is used to draw blood, and on a routine basis, according to agency policy. Depending on the type of CVC, a line that is not being used has to be flushed as often as once a day or as frequently as once a week, depending on the type of device and agency policy. A CVC should be flushed with at least 10 ml of normal saline (NS) whenever it is irrigated. Some agencies advocate the use of, at least, 3–5 ml of 100 U/ml heparin instilled after the saline, to maintain patency of the line (except for Groshong® CVCs).

The method employed to irrigate a CVC is the pulsatile, push-pause method. The volume of heparin (100 U/ml) is dictated by manufacturer guidelines and agency policy or by medical orders specific to the patient's needs. Failure to use the pulsatile, push-pause method of flushing may result in catheter occlusion.

The Groshong® tip CVC is a soft, medical-grade silicone catheter with a closed-end, atraumatic rounded tip. It is available as a tunneled, long-term CVC that has the SureCuff® Tissue Ingrowth Cuff, which is positioned in the tunnel to promote adherence to tissue and secure the catheter in place. It also is available as a noncuffed (nontunneled) short-term-use CVC and peripherally inserted central catheter (PICC).

The Groshong® tip differs from other CVCs (which are open-ended) in that it has a patented three-position, pressure-sensitive valve (or valves), which allows fluids to flow in or out but stays closed when not in use, thereby reducing the need for clamping. The valve is located near the rounded, closed, radiopaque catheter tip and allows fluid infusion and blood aspiration. When not in use, the valve restricts blood backflow (bleed-back) and air embolism by remaining closed.

The Groshong® tip CVC virtually eliminates heparin flushing to maintain catheter patency, as only saline is needed after use to maintain the valve in its normal closed position. When the catheter is not in use, it has to be flushed with normal saline only every 7 days.

ACTION TAKEN	COMPLETED SUCCESSFULLY	DID NOT COMPLETE	NOTES
1. Check the physician's order.			
2. Introduce yourself to the patient.			
3. Identify the patient by checking the wristband against the doctor's order and asking the patient, if conscious, to state his/her name.			

(continues)

Skill 14 | *(continued)*

Name _____ Date _____ Instructor _____

ACTION TAKEN	COMPLETED SUCCESSFULLY	DID NOT COMPLETE	NOTES
4. Verify the patient's allergy status.			
5. Explain the proposed procedure in terms the patient can understand.			
6. Carry out proper hand hygiene.			
7. Gather equipment and have all necessary saline and heparin drawn up before beginning the procedure.			
8. Provide for the patient's privacy.			
9. Set up equipment.			
10. Put on gloves.			
11. Cleanse the central venous catheter cap with 70% isopropyl alcohol followed by povidone-iodine (or per agency policy). Allow each solution to air-dry.			
12. Attach to the CVC a syringe containing normal saline.			
13. Instruct the patient to perform the Valsalva maneuver, and open the CVC clamp.			
14. Flush the line with normal saline. Use the pulsatile, push–pause method. Clamp the line.			
15. Attach the syringe with the heparin.			
16. Instruct the patient to perform the Valsalva maneuver, and open the CVC clamp.			

Skill 14 | *(continued)*

Name _____ Date _____ Instructor _____

ACTION TAKEN	COMPLETED SUCCESSFULLY	DID NOT COMPLETE	NOTES
17. Flush the line with the heparin, and clamp the line while infusing the last 0.5 ml of solution.			
18. Document the procedure.			

Skill 15 | Changing Injection Caps on the CVC

Name _____ Date _____ Instructor _____

Approximate Time to Complete the Skill: 5–6 minutes/cap

Overview of the Skill

An injection cap is a small device with a resealable rubber cap that is used to cap a central venous catheter (CVC) port. It is accessible by puncture with a needle or, if designed for a needleless system, with a blunt-tipped spike.

Injection caps have to be changed routinely to prevent coring after repeated needle access. Large-bore needles never should be used to access a cap, because coring can occur. Coring may cause a small segment of the cap material to enter the bloodstream and create an embolus. Only a 20–25-gauge, 1-inch needle should be used to penetrate the cap. The cap on a CVC is typically changed at least every 7 days—more frequently if the line is accessed repeatedly. The cap is to be replaced whenever a CVC dressing is changed. For a multi-lumen line, all caps should be changed simultaneously.

A Leur-Lok® that is built into the cap must be assessed regularly to ensure that the connection is secure. This is important in preventing entry of air (and the predisposition to air embolism), fluid leakage, and introduction of microorganisms into the line.

With the use of needleless systems, which are commonly used, a blunt-end device with a reflux valve or Luer-Lok® valve is used instead of an injection cap. Before changing an injection cap, the nurse always should refer to specific information from the manufacturer.

ACTION TAKEN	COMPLETED SUCCESSFULLY	DID NOT COMPLETE	NOTES
1. Check the physician's order.			
2. Verify the schedule.			
3. Introduce yourself to the patient.			
4. Identify the patient by checking the wristband against the doctor's order and asking the patient, if conscious, to state his/her name.			
5. Verify the patient's allergy status.			
6. Explain the proposed procedure in terms the patient can understand.			
7. Gather all necessary equipment.			
8. Carry out proper hand hygiene.			
9. Verify the schedule for replacing the injection cap.			
10. Provide for the patient's privacy.			

Skill 15 | *(continued)*

Name _____ Date _____ Instructor _____

ACTION TAKEN	COMPLETED SUCCESSFULLY	DID NOT COMPLETE	NOTES
11. Instruct the patient to position the head to the side opposite the CVC insertion site.			
12. Aseptically open the package containing the injection cap.			
13. Prime the injection cap with normal saline per the manufacturer's guidelines.			
14. Don gloves.			
15. Close the slide clamp on the catheter pigtail.			
16. Grasp the hub of the pigtail with your nondominant hand and the injection cap with the other hand. (For enhanced traction, use 2 × 2-inch gauze [optional] to hold the hub and injection cap.)			
17. Instruct the patient to perform the Valsalva maneuver and, while the patient is holding the breath, quickly twist off (counter-clockwise direction) and remove the used cap and connect the new cap. Be sure the Luer-Lok® is secure (clockwise twisting direction).			
18. Instruct the patient to resume his/her usual breathing pattern.			
19. Open the slide clamp.			

(continues)

Skill 15 | (continued)

Name _____ Date _____ Instructor _____

ACTION TAKEN	COMPLETED SUCCESSFULLY	DID NOT COMPLETE	NOTES
20. Prep the top of the injection cap (or remove the sterile cap from the needleless system, if applicable), first with the 70% isopropyl alcohol, then with the CHG or povidone-iodine (or per agency policy).			
21. Attach to the Luer-Lok® connection the 10-ml syringe containing the normal saline. Aspirate to confirm placement of the CVC. (There is not always a blood return.) When aspirating, allow the blood to flow only a short distance into the pigtail. Do not aspirate blood back into the syringe.			
22. Inject 4.5 ml of NS with a continuous forward motion on the plunger, exerting the pulsatile flush movement on the plunger. If encountering resistance while injecting, do not exert pressure on the CVC by exerting force on the syringe plunger. Make no further attempts to flush. *Notify the physician.*			

Skill 15 | *(continued)*

Name _____ Date _____ Instructor _____

ACTION TAKEN	COMPLETED SUCCESSFULLY	DID NOT COMPLETE	NOTES
23. Attach the 10-ml syringe containing the heparin solution to the Luer-Lok® connection. Inject the 2.5 ml of heparin solution (except for Groshong® CVCs), injecting only part of the last 0.5 ml, following the guidelines for needle and needleless systems.			
24. Change all other caps, if present, following the same guidelines.			
25. Discard in the sharps container the used injection cap and any syringes/needles used.			
26. Remove gloves.			
27. Carry out proper hand hygiene.			
28. Document the procedure.			

Skill 16 | Heparin-Locking the CVC

Name _____ Date _____ Instructor _____

Approximate Time to Complete the Skill: 5–6 minutes/pigtail

Overview of the Skill

A central venous catheter (CVC) can be heparinized per physician order to maintain patency. For a multi-lumen CVC, the pigtails of each lumen should be heparinized, if ordered. For any cannula not in use, heparin flushing should be done every 8–12 hours following the institution-approved procedure. The strength of heparin solution used is usually 100 U/ml but may range from 10–1000 U/ml, depending on the patient's condition and the agency's policy.

ACTION TAKEN	COMPLETED SUCCESSFULLY	DID NOT COMPLETE	NOTES
1. Check the physician's order.			
2. Verify the schedule.			
3. Introduce yourself to the patient.			
4. Identify the patient by checking the wristband against the doctor's order and asking the patient, if conscious, to state his/her name.			
5. Verify the patient's allergy status.			
6. Explain the proposed procedure in terms the patient can understand.			
7. Gather all necessary equipment.			
8. Carry out proper hand hygiene.			
9. Verify the schedule for replacing the injection cap.			
10. Provide for the patient's privacy.			
11. Instruct the patient to position the head to the side opposite the CVC insertion site.			
12. Aseptically open the package containing the injection cap.			

Skill 16 | *(continued)*

Name _____ Date _____ Instructor _____

ACTION TAKEN	COMPLETED SUCCESSFULLY	DID NOT COMPLETE	NOTES
13. Prime the injection cap with normal saline per manufacturer's guidelines.			
14. Don gloves.			
15. Close the slide clamp on the catheter pigtail.			
16. Grasp the hub of the pigtail with your nondominant hand and the injection cap with the other hand. (For enhanced traction, use 2 × 2-inch gauze [optional] to hold the hub and injection cap.)			
17. Instruct the patient to perform the Valsalva maneuver and, as the patient is holding the breath, quickly twist off (counter-clockwise direction) and remove the used cap and connect the new cap. Be sure the Luer-Lok® is secure (clockwise twisting direction).			
18. Instruct the patient to resume his/her usual breathing pattern.			
19. Open the slide clamp.			
20. Prep the top of the injection cap (or remove the sterile cap from the needleless system, if applicable), first with the 70% isopropyl alcohol, then with the CHG or povidone-iodine (or per agency policy).			

(continues)

Skill 16 | *(continued)*

Name _____ Date _____ Instructor _____

ACTION TAKEN	COMPLETED SUCCESSFULLY	DID NOT COMPLETE	NOTES
21. Attach the 10-ml syringe containing the normal saline to the Luer-Lok® connection. Aspirate to confirm placement of the CVC. (There may not always be a blood return.) When aspirating, allow the blood to flow only a short distance into the pigtail. Do not aspirate blood back into the syringe.			
22. Inject 4.5 ml of NS with a continuous forward motion on the plunger, exerting the pulsatile flush movement on the plunger. If encountering resistance while injecting, do not exert pressure on the CVC by exerting force on the syringe plunger. Do not make further attempts to flush. *Notify the physician*.			
23. Attach to the Luer-Lok® connection the 10-ml syringe containing the heparin solution. Inject the 2.5 ml of heparin solution (except Groshong® CVCs), injecting only part of the last 0.5 ml, following the guidelines for needle and needleless systems.			
24. Change all other caps, if present, following the same guidelines.			

Skill 16 | *(continued)*

Name _____ Date _____ Instructor _____

ACTION TAKEN	COMPLETED SUCCESSFULLY	DID NOT COMPLETE	NOTES
25. Discard in the sharps container the used injection cap and any syringes/needles used.			
26. Remove gloves.			
27. Carry out proper hand hygiene.			
28. Document the procedure in the Medication Administration Record (MAR). In the nurse's notes, report any problems encountered.			

Skill 17 | Drawing Blood from the CVC

Name _____ Date _____ Instructor _____

Approximate Time to Complete the Skill: 10 minutes

Overview of the Skill

Patients who have a central venous catheter (CVC) may have blood drawn from the catheter. This eliminates the need for repeated venipuncture, making the patient more comfortable and reducing the risk for injury.

Some sources state that certain blood tests should not be run on samples taken from an IV that has been used to infuse certain medications. Peak and trough levels for antibiotics may be more accurate if drawn peripherally rather than from the central line used for administration. This may not be possible for a patient with poor peripheral access.

In most agencies, only registered nurses who are trained to work with central lines and care for patients who have them are authorized to draw blood specimens from CVCs.

An ALERT sign, stating that only RNs are to draw blood, is placed over the head of the patient's bed and on the chart to prevent needless attempts at peripheral blood sampling.

ACTION TAKEN	COMPLETED SUCCESSFULLY	DID NOT COMPLETE	NOTES
1. Check the physician's order.			
2. Check the orders for the lab work.			
3. Introduce yourself to the patient.			
4. Identify the patient by checking the wristband against the doctor's order and asking the patient, if conscious, to state his/her name.			
5. Verify the patient's allergy status.			
6. Explain the proposed procedure in terms the patient can understand.			
7. Carry out proper hand hygiene.			
8. Gather equipment and have all necessary heparin and saline drawn up prior to beginning the procedure.			
9. Provide for the patient's privacy.			
10. Set up equipment.			
11. Put on gloves.			

Skill 17 | *(continued)*

Name _____ Date _____ Instructor _____

ACTION TAKEN	COMPLETED SUCCESSFULLY	DID NOT COMPLETE	NOTES
12. If an infusion is running and the patient has a single-lumen CVC: a. Close the slide clamp on the pigtail. b. Instruct the patient to perform the Valsalva maneuver, then quickly disconnect the administration set tubing from the pigtail, cap the pigtail with the injection cap, and cap the distal end of the administration set with the sterile cap.			
13. For multi-lumen CVCs, use the proximal lumen to draw blood, and for one full minute turn off all electrolyte and glucose-containing infusates that are infusing into other lumens.			
14. Prep the injection cap of the pigtail with the alcohol, followed by the 2% CHG or iodophor (or per agency policy).			
15. Attach a 10-ml saline-filled syringe. Open the slide clamp and ascertain placement and patency of the CVC, then vigorously flush with 10 ml of NS using the pulsatile, push-pause method. Clamp.			

(continues)

Skill 17 | (continued)

Name _____ Date _____ Instructor _____

ACTION TAKEN	COMPLETED SUCCESSFULLY	DID NOT COMPLETE	NOTES
16. Attach the vacuum container to the injection cap. Unclamp.			
17. Draw 5 to 10 ml of blood into the discard tube. (The first flow of fluid into the tube will be clear, as it is the fluid that is in the pigtail.)	`		
18. Quickly insert and fill the required blood collection tube, then close the slide clamp on the pigtail and remove the vacuum container collecting device. Clamp.			
19. Prep the injection cap, open the slide clamp, and vigorously flush the line with at least 20 ml of NS to remove any residual blood. Clamp.			
20. Reconnect the infusion line, and unclamp so the infusion may run (or unclamp, heparin-lock the pigtail, then clamp).			
21. As soon as the blood draw is complete and the integrity of the CVC is ensured, label the blood tubes and deliver the sample to the laboratory.			
22. Dispose of used equipment and carry out proper hand hygiene.			
23. Document the procedure.			

Skill 18 | The POP Method

Name _____ Date _____ Instructor _____

Approximate Time to Complete the Skill: 10–15 minutes

Overview of the Skill

Central lines can become occluded for several reasons. An occlusion caused by clots, lipids, or some precipitates may be cleared using the POP method. This method uses negative pressure to clear the line by pulling the clot or residue back into the syringe. Do not use this method with polyurethane catheters.

ACTION TAKEN	COMPLETED SUCCESSFULLY	DID NOT COMPLETE	NOTES
1. Check the physician's order.			
2. Introduce yourself to the patient.			
3. Identify the patient by checking the wristband against the doctor's order and asking the patient, if conscious, to state his/her name.			
4. Verify the patient's allergy status.			
5. Explain the proposed procedure in terms the patient can understand.			
6. Carry out proper hand hygiene.			
7. Gather all necessary equipment.			
8. Follow the medical order or agency policy regarding clearing occluded CVCs.			
9. Provide for the patient's privacy.			
10. Set up equipment.			
11. Put on gloves.			
12. Cleanse the central venous catheter cap with 70% isopropyl alcohol followed by 2% CHG or povidone-iodine (or per agency policy). Allow each solution to air-dry.			

(continues)

Skill 18 | *(continued)*

Name _____ Date _____ Instructor _____

ACTION TAKEN	COMPLETED SUCCESSFULLY	DID NOT COMPLETE	NOTES
13. Instruct the patient to perform the Valsalva maneuver. Then open the CVC clamp.			
14. Disconnect the catheter cap or IV infusion line (covering the tubing end with a sterile cap) and attach to the catheter hub the 20-ml syringe containing the 5 ml of NS. Instruct the patient to breathe normally.			
15. Open the slide clamp.			
16. Pull back on the syringe plunger to the 15-ml mark and let go of the plunger. A popping sound will result.			
17. Repeat the maneuver several times in rapid succession. (Follow the same procedure for the 3 French catheter, but pull back to the 10-ml mark on the syringe.)			
18. Ask the patient to perform the Valsalva maneuver until told to discontinue it.			
19. Remove the syringe and attach the syringe filled with the 20 ml of NS to the hub (or smaller syringe for smaller CVC). Instruct the patient to breathe normally.			
20. Open the slide clamp.			

Skill 18 | *(continued)*

Name _____ Date _____ Instructor _____

ACTION TAKEN	COMPLETED SUCCESSFULLY	DID NOT COMPLETE	NOTES
21. Attempt to flush. If no resistance is felt, flush vigorously, using the pulsatile, push-pause method.			
22. Close the slide clamp.			
23. Ask the patient to perform the Valsalva maneuver until told to discontinue it.			
24. Attach the sterile injection cap to the catheter hub and heparin-lock the catheter or attach the IV line to the catheter hub and regulate the infusion.			
24. Instruct the patient to breathe normally.			
26. Document in the nurse's notes.			

Skill 19 | The Positive Pressure Method

Name _____ Date _____ Instructor _____

Approximate Time to Complete the Skill: 15 minutes plus time allowed for declotting agent to work

Overview of the Skill

When an occlusion cannot be cleared using the POP method, use of a thrombolytic agent can help. For this method, a physician's order is required. Agency policy and the physician's order must be followed precisely.

ACTION TAKEN	COMPLETED SUCCESSFULLY	DID NOT COMPLETE	NOTES
1. Check the physician's order.			
2. Introduce yourself to the patient.			
3. Identify the patient by checking the wristband against the doctor's order and asking the patient, if conscious, to state his/her name.			
4. Verify the patient's allergy status.			
5. Explain the proposed procedure in terms the patient can understand.			
6. Gather all necessary equipment.			
7. Carry out proper hand hygiene.			
8. Follow the medical order or agency policy regarding clearing occluded CVCs.			
9. Provide for the patient's privacy.			
10. Set up equipment.			
11. Put on gloves.			
12. Cleanse the central venous catheter cap with 70% isopropyl alcohol followed by 2% CHG or povidone-iodine (or per agency policy). Allow each solution to air-dry.			

Skill 19 | *(continued)*

Name _____ Date _____ Instructor _____

ACTION TAKEN	COMPLETED SUCCESSFULLY	DID NOT COMPLETE	NOTES
13. If the CVC is connected to an infusion line, close the slide clamp, and instruct the patient to perform the Valsalva maneuver. Disconnect the catheter cap or IV infusion line (covering the tubing end with a sterile cap) and attach the empty syringe to the CVC hub. Instruct the patient to breathe normally.			
14. Open the slide clamp and attempt to aspirate. a. If successful, withdraw the clots/residue(s), close the slide clamp, detach the syringe, and proceed to the next step. b. If aspiration is unsuccessful, close the slide clamp, have the patient perform the Valsalva maneuver, then detach the syringe and proceed to step 17.			

(continues)

Skill 19 | *(continued)*

Name _____ Date _____ Instructor _____

ACTION TAKEN	COMPLETED SUCCESSFULLY	DID NOT COMPLETE	NOTES
15. Attach the syringe containing the 10 ml (or 20 ml) of NS and flush vigorously, using the pulsatile, push-pause method. Then do one of the following: a. Close the slide clamp, have the patient perform the Valsalva maneuver, attach the syringe with the heparin flush, have the patient breathe normally, open the slide clamp, heparin-lock the line, and close the slide clamp. OR b. Close the slide clamp, have the patient perform the Valsalva maneuver, connect the IV tubing to the CVC hub, have the patient breathe normally, unclamp, and regulate the infusion.			
16. Document the procedure.			
17. Attach the syringe containing the prescribed amount of thrombolytic agent (or other declotting agent) and have the patient breathe normally.			
18. Open the slide clamp.			

Skill 19 | *(continued)*

Name _____ Date _____ Instructor _____

ACTION TAKEN	COMPLETED SUCCESSFULLY	DID NOT COMPLETE	NOTES
19. Slowly and gently inject the declotting agent into the catheter, using a push-pull motion. If strong resistance is encountered, do not force the entire amount into the catheter.			
20. Leave the syringe attached to the catheter for 30 to 90 minutes (or per physician's order or agency policy), and do not attempt to aspirate during this time.			
21. After the prescribed amount of time, attempt to aspirate. a. If unsuccessful, repeat the procedure or notify the physician, depending on agency policy. b. If patency is restored, aspirate 5 ml to 10 ml of blood.			
22. Close the clamp.			
23. Have the patient perform the Valsalva maneuver, attach the 20-ml NS-filled syringe, have the patient breathe normally, and open the clamp.			
24. Flush the line vigorously, using the pulsatile, push-pause method, then close the slide clamp.			
25. Attach the injection cap and heparin-lock the catheter or attach the IV line and regulate the infusion.			
26. Document the procedure.			

Skill 20 | The Stopcock-Negative Pressure Method

Name _____ Date _____ Instructor _____

Approximate Time to Complete the Skill: 20 minutes plus prescribed time for declotting agent to work

Overview of the Skill

The purpose of the stopcock-negative pressure method for clearing an occluded central line is to use negative pressure to create a vacuum in which to instill the declotting agent. This will decrease the amount of pressure on the central-line cannula when administering the agent, which will prevent possible rupture of the catheter.

ACTION TAKEN	COMPLETED SUCCESSFULLY	DID NOT COMPLETE	NOTES
1. Check the physician's order.			
2. Introduce yourself to the patient.			
3. Identify the patient by checking the wristband against the doctor's order and asking the patient, if conscious, to state his/her name.			
4. Verify the patient's allergy status.			
5. Explain the proposed procedure in terms the patient can understand.			
6. Gather all necessary equipment.			
7. Carry out proper hand hygiene.			
8. Follow the medical order or agency policy regarding clearing occluded CVCs.			
9. Provide for the patient's privacy.			
10. Set up equipment.			
11. Put on gloves.			
12. Cleanse the central venous catheter cap with 70% isopropyl alcohol followed by 2% CHG or povidone-iodine (or per agency policy). Allow each solution to air-dry.			

Skill 20 | *(continued)*

Name _____ Date _____ Instructor _____

ACTION TAKEN	COMPLETED SUCCESSFULLY	DID NOT COMPLETE	NOTES
13. If the CVC is connected to an infusion line, close the slide clamp, have the patient perform the Valsalva maneuver, disconnect the catheter cap or IV infusion line (covering the tubing end with a sterile cap), and attach the empty syringe to the CVC hub. Instruct the patient to breathe normally. Turn the three-way stopcock to the "off" position before it is attached to the CVC hub.			
14. Close the slide clamp, instruct the patient to perform the Valsalva maneuver, attach the closed stop-cock to the CVC hub, and open the CVC clamp. Instruct the patient to breathe normally.			
15. Cleanse one port of the stopcock with alcohol and 2% CHG or povidone-iodine (if sterility has been breached), and attach it to the empty 20-ml syringe.			
16. Cleanse the other port of the stop-cock, as before (if sterility has been breached), and attach it to the 20-ml syringe containing the declotting agent.			

(continues)

Skill 20 | *(continued)*

Name _____ Date _____ Instructor _____

ACTION TAKEN	COMPLETED SUCCESSFULLY	DID NOT COMPLETE	NOTES
17. Turn off the stopcock to the syringe containing the declotting agent and open it to the empty 20-ml syringe.			
18. Open the slide clamp on the CVC.			
19. Gently aspirate the CVC until the plunger is pulled back to the 15-ml marking.			
20. With the plunger retracted to the 15-ml mark, turn off the stopcock to the plunger-aspirated syringe.			
21. Open the stopcock ("on" position) to the syringe that contains the declotting agent.			
22. Turn the stopcock to the "off" position, leaving the declotting agent in the CVC lumen for the prescribed time (per manufacturer/ agency/physician recommendations).			
23. Open the stopcock and aspirate for a blood return. If blood is returned, aspirate a waste volume of 5 to 10 ml. If aspiration is unsuccessful, repeat the procedure or notify the physician, depending on agency policy. Close the catheter clamp.			

Skill 20 | *(continued)*

Name _____ Date _____ Instructor _____

ACTION TAKEN	COMPLETED SUCCESSFULLY	DID NOT COMPLETE	NOTES
24. Have the patient perform the Valsalva maneuver. Then remove the stopcock and attach the 20-ml syringe containing the NS to the catheter hub. Instruct the patient to breathe normally.			
25. Open the catheter slide clamp and vigorously flush the catheter, using the pulsatile, push-pause method. Close the slide clamp.			
26. Have the patient perform the Valsalva maneuver. Then do one of the following: a. Open the slide clamp and attach the heparin flush syringe. Instruct the patient to breathe normally. Instill the heparin solution and close the clamp. b. After removing the syringe, connect the IV infusion line, open the slide clamp, and regulate the infusion.			
27. Document the procedure.			

Skill 21 | Removal of the CVC

Name _____ Date _____ Instructor _____

Approximate Time to Complete the Skill: 5–10 minutes

Overview of the Skill

Most agencies have a policy designating that a registered nurse may take out a nontunneled central line once the physician has written the order for removal, if approved by the state Nurse Practice Act. The removal of tunneled or implanted catheters is generally considered a medical duty.

ACTION TAKEN	COMPLETED SUCCESSFULLY	DID NOT COMPLETE	NOTES
1. Check the physician's order.			
2. Introduce yourself to the patient.			
3. Identify the patient by checking the wristband against the doctor's order and asking the patient, if conscious, to state his/her name.			
4. Verify the patient's allergy status.			
5. Explain the proposed procedure in terms the patient can understand.			
6. Gather all necessary supplies.			
7. Carry out proper hand hygiene.			
8. Provide privacy to the patient.			
9. Review with the patient the procedure for performing the Valsalva maneuver.			
10. Elevate the patient's bed level and position the bed in the Trendelenburg or flat position.			
11. Attach the plastic disposal bag to the side of the bed or overbed table, or place the plastic sheeting in close proximity to the patient.			

Skill 21 | *(continued)*

Name _____ Date _____ Instructor _____

ACTION TAKEN	COMPLETED SUCCESSFULLY	DID NOT COMPLETE	NOTES
12. Carry out proper hand hygiene.			
13. Clamp the infusion tubing and turn off the electronic infusion device (if appropriate).			
14. Close the slide clamp on the CVC.			
15. Don disposable gloves.			
16. Remove the dressing, following the guidelines for dressing removal as described in Skill 13, CVC Dressing Change and Site Care.			
17. Inspect the dressing for purulent drainage or foul odor.			
18. Discard the dressing in the plastic bag or on the plastic sheeting.			
19. Remove gloves and carry out proper hand hygiene.			
20. Place 4 × 4-inch gauze, skin antiseptics, suture-removal kit, and dressing materials in close proximity to the patient, and open them, using aseptic technique.			
21. Don sterile gloves, leaving the inside (sterile portion) of the wrapper at the bedside.			
22. Inspect the site around the cannula insertion area.			

(continues)

Skill 21 | *(continued)*

Name _____ Date _____ Instructor _____

ACTION TAKEN	COMPLETED SUCCESSFULLY	DID NOT COMPLETE	NOTES
23. Cleanse the CVC insertion site and surrounding area, including the catheter and sutures, in a concentric circle, starting at the catheter exit site. Clean first with the alcohol, repeating as needed to remove all debris. If necessary, use adhesive remover to eliminate any tape deposits. Follow with thorough cleansing using the 2% CHG or povidone-iodine, and allow the area to air-dry.			
24. Carefully clip and remove sutures while securing the CVC.			
25. Place the 4 × 4-inch sterile gauze over the CVC exit site, holding it in place with the nondominant hand.			
26. Instruct the patient to perform the Valsalva maneuver. Withdraw the CVC from the vein in one smooth, steady motion, continuing to hold the 4 × 4-inch gauze in place.			
27. Exert firm pressure over the exit site for 1 to 5 minutes after the catheter is out, and discard the catheter on the sterile inner wrapper from the gloves. Instruct the patient to breathe normally. Continue to apply pressure until any bleeding stops.			

Skill 21 | *(continued)*

Name _____ Date _____ Instructor _____

ACTION TAKEN	COMPLETED SUCCESSFULLY	DID NOT COMPLETE	NOTES
28. Apply the sterile air-occlusive dressing over the site and secure the edges so air cannot enter. The dressing is to be left in place for 24 to 72 hours.			
29. Examine the removed CVC and assess it for drainage, odor, integrity, and length. a. If there is any breach in the CVC structure, instruct the patient to maintain complete bedrest. Save the catheter and notify the physician immediately. b. If there is any drainage or foul smell, cut off the tip (2–3 inches) and place the tip portion of the CVC in a sterile specimen container for culture studies.			
30. Dispose of used equipment and carry out proper hand hygiene.			
31. Assess the dressing every 15 minutes for the first hour after removal, then hourly for the first 24 hours post-removal. The patient should maintain bedrest, as needed, until the exit site has epithelialized.			

(continues)

Skill 21 | *(continued)*

Name _____ Date _____ Instructor _____

ACTION TAKEN	COMPLETED SUCCESSFULLY	DID NOT COMPLETE	NOTES
32. Document the patient's response to CVC removal, appearance of the site, dressing regimen, and condition and length of the catheter, as well as any associated interventions.			

Skill 22 | Insertion of the Peripherally Inserted Central Catheter

Name _____ Date _____ Instructor _____

Approximate Time to Complete the Skill: 30 minutes

Overview of the Skill

A peripherally inserted central catheter (PICC) is a percutaneous single- or multi-lumen infusion line that is inserted via the large antecubital basilic or cephalic vein or the median cubital vein. Although the basilic vein is usually the first choice, each has advantages and disadvantages. The tip of the PICC is placed in the superior vena cava at the entrance to the right atrium of the heart. Nurses trained in the procedure often insert this type of central venous catheter (CVC).

Insertion of a PICC varies slightly depending on the product used. Some PICCs are inserted through a breakaway needle. After the PICC is placed, the needle is split and peeled away. Other PICCs are inserted through an over-the-needle cannula that acts as an introducer. The needle is removed, leaving a cannula in place, and the PICC is threaded through the cannula. Some PICCs have a guidewire that makes the catheter firm as it is introduced. Guidewires usually are found in larger-gauge PICCs.

PICC lines are indicated for the administration of fluids, blood or blood products, and medications in patients who lack suitable veins for repeated peripheral vascular access. If placed in the superior vena cava, PICC lines also are used to draw blood for sampling, to administer chemotherapy, and in parenteral nutrition preparations. They usually are intended for patients who require therapy from periods of 1–12 weeks or longer.

Fewer complications are associated with a PICC than with other types of CVCs. Advantages associated with PICC lines include

- avoiding the discomfort and stress affiliated with multiple peripheral sticks
- less trauma because PICC poses fewer risks than are associated with insertions in the neck and chest regions (i.e., pneumothorax and great vessel perforation)
- insertion on an outpatient basis
- reduced risk of infiltration
- lowest incidence of complications upon insertion compared to other CVCs
- decreased risk of phlebitis
- preservation of peripheral veins
- cost-effectiveness
- no age barrier.

PICC lines are contraindicated in patients

- with inadequate antecubital veins (candidates must have a peripheral antecubital vein large enough to accommodate a 14–16-gauge introducer needle)
- with preexisting skin infections
- with anatomic distortions related to injury, surgical dissection, or trauma
- with severe peripheral edema
- who require high-volume or high-pressure infusions
- who cannot change the dressing
- who do heavy lifting
- whose lifestyles or occupations involve being in water.

ACTION TAKEN	COMPLETED SUCCESSFULLY	DID NOT COMPLETE	NOTES
1. Check the physician's order and institutional policy regarding insertion of a PICC.			
2. Introduce yourself to the patient.			

(continues)

Skill 22 | *(continued)*

Name _____ Date _____ Instructor _____

ACTION TAKEN	COMPLETED SUCCESSFULLY	DID NOT COMPLETE	NOTES
3. Identify the patient by checking the wristband against the doctor's order and asking the patient, if conscious, to state his/her name.			
4. Verify the patient's allergy status.			
5. Explain the proposed procedure in terms the patient can understand.			
6. Obtain the patient's consent for the procedure.			
7. Gather all necessary equipment.			
8. Carry out proper hand hygiene.			
9. Provide for the patient's privacy.			
10. Apply a tourniquet to the patient's arm and assess the arm for an appropriate insertion site. Remove the tourniquet.			
11. Measure the amount of line that will be needed according to agency policy, and write down that number.			
12. Wash the patient's arm with soap and water 6 inches above and below the insertion site; dry thoroughly.			
13. Position the patient flat with the arm extended at a 90-degree angle.			

Skill 22 | *(continued)*

Name _____ Date _____ Instructor _____

ACTION TAKEN	COMPLETED SUCCESSFULLY	DID NOT COMPLETE	NOTES
14. Carry out proper hand hygiene and open the PICC kit using sterile procedure. Drop any additional supplies on the sterile field.			
15. Place the under-drape under the patient's arm and shoulder area.			
16. Don a mask, sterile gloves, and sterile gown. Put a mask on the patient.			
17. Prepare three 10-ml syringes with normal saline.			
18. Remove the catheter from the tray and examine it; be sure the guidewire is straight.			
19. Prime the catheter with normal saline, and place the sterile measuring tape alongside the catheter.			
20. a. For a closed-ended catheter: Measure the distance from the tip of the catheter to where it will exit the body, and mark it. b. For an open-ended catheter: Measure the distance from the exit site to where the tip of the catheter will lie in the vessel.			

(continues)

Skill 22 | *(continued)*

Name _____ Date _____ Instructor _____

ACTION TAKEN	COMPLETED SUCCESSFULLY	DID NOT COMPLETE	NOTES
Note this marking, and allow for the distance of the catheter that will extend out of the arm. Retract the guidewire to where the catheter tip will be cut, cut the tip straight across, advance the guidewire to within $\frac{1}{8}$ to $\frac{1}{4}$ inch of the tip, and bend the guidewire at a 90-degree angle at the external end of the device.			
21. Prime the catheter connector.			
22. Prep the insertion site first, using three alcohol swabsticks and then three 2% aqueous chlorhexidine gluconate or iodophor swabsticks. Work outward in a concentric circle. Allow each solution to dry completely before proceeding to the next step.			
23. Place sterile drapes around the insertion site.			
24. Apply the tourniquet; for most patients this should be above the elbow.			
25. Remove the gloves used for preparation, and apply a second set of sterile gloves.			
26. Anesthetize the insertion site.			
27. Hold the skin taut below the insertion site.			

Skill 22 | *(continued)*

Name _____ Date _____ Instructor _____

ACTION TAKEN	COMPLETED SUCCESSFULLY	DID NOT COMPLETE	NOTES
28. Perform the venipuncture holding the introducer needle at a 30-degree angle with the bevel up.			
29. Look for a blood return in the flash-back chamber, then slowly advance the introducer needle a fraction of an inch more so the sheath is in the vein.			
30. Remove the tourniquet.			
31. Maintain the stability of the introducer and advance it.			
32. Observe the pattern of blood flow.			
33. Remove the needle from the introducer, leaving the intro-ducer in place.			
34. Thread the PICC into the vein through the introducer to the depth determined by previous measurements. Use a steady, moderate rate of passage.			
35. Hold pressure over the insertion site until bleeding stops.			
36. Cleanse the insertion site of all blood.			

(continues)

Skill 22 | *(continued)*

Name _____ Date _____ Instructor _____

ACTION TAKEN	COMPLETED SUCCESSFULLY	DID NOT COMPLETE	NOTES
37. Remove the guidewire by spreading the fingers of one hand over the length of the catheter outside the insertion site and pressing down gently while grasping the hub of the guidewire with the opposite hand and pulling it parallel to the skin with a slow, steady motion.			
38. Remove the introducer catheter from the PICC while applying pressure above the insertion site.			
39. Cut the PICC so approximately 10 cm remain extending from the insertion site.			
40. Insert the connector into the catheter, and apply a suture wing.			
41. Using a 10-ml syringe of saline aspirate to confirm placement of the catheter tip, flush, using the pulsatile, push-pause method.			
42. Apply an injection cap.			
43. Heparinize the injection cap.			
44. Place a 2 × 2-inch folded gauze over the insertion site, and place a transparent dressing over the gauze for the first 24 hours.			

Skill 22 | *(continued)*

Name _____ Date _____ Instructor _____

ACTION TAKEN	COMPLETED SUCCESSFULLY	DID NOT COMPLETE	NOTES
45. Label the insertion site with date, time, length and gauge of catheter, and your initials.			
46. Remove gloves, gown, and mask, and dispose of all materials in the proper waste receptacle.			
47. Carry out proper hand hygiene.			
48. Document the procedure.			
49. Be sure catheter placement is verified with a chest x-ray.			
50. Change dressing in 24 hours. Assess for swelling, drainage, and tenderness. Assess for migration of the catheter by checking the length of the catheter.			

Skill 23 | PICC Dressing Change and Site Care

Name _____ Date _____ Instructor _____

Approximate Time to Complete the Skill: 10 minutes

Overview of the Skill

A peripherally inserted central catheter (PICC) is a catheter inserted in a basilic or cephalic vein in the antecubital fossa with the tip of the catheter in the superior vena cava at the entrance to the right atrium of the heart. Because of the PICC's position in the mainstream of circulation, care must be taken to prevent the entry of microorganisms at the entrance site. This is accomplished by changing the dressing properly and observing the site closely.

Although gauze dressings are still considered acceptable, the most common type of dressing used is a transparent semipermeable dressing. If a gauze dressing is used, it must be changed when the tubing is changed. Use of gauze dressing also prevents observation of the infusion site without removing the dressing. If the dressing is partially removed to examine the site, it should be changed to prevent the introduction of microorganisms. Any dressing that becomes soiled or loosened should be changed.

A transparent semipermeable dressing allows observation of the infusion site without removing the dressing. This type of dressing should be changed every 7 days.

ACTION TAKEN	COMPLETED SUCCESSFULLY	DID NOT COMPLETE	NOTES
1. Check the physician's order and institutional policy regarding a PICC dressing change.			
2. Introduce yourself to the patient.			
3. Identify the patient by checking the wristband against the doctor's order and asking the patient, if conscious, to state his/her name.			
4. Verify the patient's allergy status.			
5. Explain the proposed procedure in terms the patient can understand.			
6. Gather all necessary equipment.			
7. Carry out proper hand hygiene.			
8. Provide for the patient's privacy.			
9. Put on the mask and assist the patient to put on a mask as well.			
10. Don disposable gloves.			

Skill 23 | *(continued)*

Name _____ Date _____ Instructor _____

ACTION TAKEN	COMPLETED SUCCESSFULLY	DID NOT COMPLETE	NOTES
11. Instruct the patient to turn his/her head in the direction opposite of the insertion site and not to move until the procedure is complete.			
12. Using the stretch method, remove the old dressing, being careful not to dislodge the catheter. Note any abnormalities.			
13. Remove gloves and carry out proper hand hygiene.			
14. Open the central line dressing pack and apply sterile gloves.			
15. Pick up the sterile drape and drape the patient below the insertion site.			
16. Cleanse the site with each of three alcohol swabs. Cleansing should occur in a circular motion, starting at the center of the insertion site and spiraling outward. Allow the alcohol to dry between swabs.			
17. Cleanse the site with each of three 2% CHG or povidone-iodine swabs. Cleanse in a circular motion, starting at the center of the insertion site and spiraling outward. Allow the area to air-dry.			

(continues)

Skill 23 | *(continued)*

Name _____ Date _____ Instructor _____

ACTION TAKEN	COMPLETED SUCCESSFULLY	DID NOT COMPLETE	NOTES
18. Apply either a transparent semipermeable dressing or a gauze dressing over the site, with the insertion site in the center. If using a gauze dressing, tape over all the gauze and edges.			
19. Note the date, time, length of the catheter outside insertion site, and total length of catheter; then initial the dressing, being careful not to prevent visual inspection of the insertion site.			
20. Dispose of used equipment and carry out proper hand hygiene.			
21. Document the procedure.			

Skill 24 | PICC Injection Cap Changes

Name _____ Date _____ Instructor _____

Approximate Time to Complete the Skill: 5–6 minutes per cap

Overview of the Skill

An injection cap is a small device with a resealable rubber cap, used to cap an IV catheter. It can be punctured by a needle, or if designed for needleless systems, with a blunt-tipped spike.

Injection caps have to be changed routinely to prevent coring after repeated uses or when large-bore needles are used. Coring can allow a small segment of the cap material to enter into the bloodstream, creating an embolus. Routine changes of the injection cap will help eliminate this problem. Injection caps on peripherally inserted central catheters (PICCs) usually are changed a minimum of every 7 days, more often if the line is accessed frequently. Caps usually are changed when changing the PICC dressing. When changing the caps on a multi-lumen line, all caps should be changed at the same time.

Injection caps are attached by a Luer-Lok® connection. The connection has to be checked frequently to ensure that it has not loosened and that it will not allow leakage and the introduction of microorganisms into the line.

Before changing an injection cap, the nurse always should refer to any specific information from the manufacturer.

ACTION TAKEN	COMPLETED SUCCESSFULLY	DID NOT COMPLETE	NOTES
1. Check the physician's order and institutional policy regarding how to change a PICC injection cap.			
2. Check to be sure the cap has to be changed.			
3. Introduce yourself to the patient.			
4. Identify the patient by checking the wristband against the doctor's order and asking the patient, if conscious, to state his/her name.			
5. Verify the patient's allergy status.			
6. Explain the proposed procedure in terms the patient can understand.			
7. Obtain the patient's consent for the procedure.			
8. Gather all necessary equipment.			
9. Carry out proper hand hygiene.			
10. Provide for the patient's privacy.			

(continues)

Skill 24 | *(continued)*

Name _____ Date _____ Instructor _____

ACTION TAKEN	COMPLETED SUCCESSFULLY	DID NOT COMPLETE	NOTES
11. Draw up 1 cc of normal saline in the syringe. Flush all air out of the injection cap.			
12. If the PICC cannot be clamped, place the patient in a supine position.			
13. Put on the gloves.			
14. Thoroughly cleanse the connection site between the injection cap and the PICC with the alcohol swab. Allow the site to air-dry.			
15. Instruct the patient to turn his/her head away from the PICC during the procedure.			
16. If not contraindicated, clamp the PICC. If clamping is contraindicated, instruct the patient to perform the Valsalva maneuver until instructed to stop.			
17. Remove the old injection cap by twisting the cap to the left.			
18. Add the new injection cap by twisting the cap to the right. Instruct the patient to breathe normally again.			
19. Change all other caps, if present, following the same procedure.			
20. Dispose of all used equipment and carry out proper hand hygiene.			
21. Document the procedure.			

Skill 25 | Flushing the PICC

Name _____ Date _____ Instructor _____

Approximate Time to Complete the Skill: 5 minutes

Overview of the Skill

Routine flushing of a peripherally inserted central catheter (PICC) is an extremely important maintenance measure to ensure patency of the line. PICCs should be flushed routinely, using normal saline, followed by heparin (except for Groshong® PICCs), based on agency policy guidelines. The flushing volume is dictated by agency policy but usually is 5–10 ml (the Groshong® PICC requires 5 ml). Open-ended PICC lines must have the last 0.5 ml of heparin instilled using the end-positive pressure method to prevent blood reflux.

A PICC is to be flushed or irrigated

- whenever the line is locked
- after every blood draw
- following intermittent administration of medication
- following transfusion of blood or blood product
- following total or peripheral parenteral nutrition.

ACTION TAKEN	COMPLETED SUCCESSFULLY	DID NOT COMPLETE	NOTES
1. Check the physician's order and institutional policy regarding PICC line flushes.			
2. Introduce yourself to the patient.			
3. Identify the patient by checking the wristband against the doctor's order and asking the patient, if conscious, to state his/her name.			
4. Verify the patient's allergy status.			
5. Explain the proposed procedure in terms the patient can understand.			
6. Gather all necessary equipment.			
7. Carry out proper hand hygiene.			
8. Provide for the patient's privacy.			
9. Set up equipment.			
10. Put on gloves.			

(continues)

Skill 25 | *(continued)*

Name _____ Date _____ Instructor _____

ACTION TAKEN	COMPLETED SUCCESSFULLY	DID NOT COMPLETE	NOTES
11. Cleanse the central venous catheter cap with 70% isopropyl alcohol followed by 2% CHG or povidone-iodine (or per agency policy). Allow each solution to air-dry.			
12. Attach the syringe containing normal saline to PICC.			
13. Instruct the patient to perform the Valsalva maneuver. Then open the PICC clamp and flush the line with normal saline, using the pulsatile, push-pause method. Clamp the line. Instruct the patient to breathe normally.			
14. Attach the syringe with the heparin.			
15. Instruct the patient to perform the Valsalva maneuver. Open the PICC clamp, and flush the line with the heparin. Clamp the line while infusing the last 0.5 ml of solution. Instruct the patient to breathe normally.			
16. Dispose of all used equipment and carry out proper hand hygiene.			
17. Document the procedure.			

Skill 26 | Drawing Blood from the PICC

Name _____ Date _____ Instructor _____

Approximate Time to Complete the Skill: 10 minutes

Overview of the Skill

The ability to draw blood samples from a peripherally inserted central catheter (PICC) line may depend on the catheter size. A 4 French, 18-gauge, or greater usually is required for successful blood sampling. Patients who have a central venous catheter (CVC) may have blood drawn from the catheter. This eliminates the need for repeated venipuncture, making the patient more comfortable and at less risk for injury.

Note: Some sources state that certain blood tests should not be run on samples taken from an IV that has been used to infuse certain medications. Peak and trough levels for antibiotics may be more accurate if drawn peripherally rather than from the central line used for administration. This may not be possible for a patient with poor peripheral access.

In most agencies, only registered nurses who are trained to work with central lines and care for patients who have them are authorized to draw blood specimens from PICCs. An ALERT sign, stating that RNs only are to draw blood, is placed over the head of the patient's bed and on the chart to prevent needless attempts at peripheral blood sampling.

ACTION TAKEN	COMPLETED SUCCESSFULLY	DID NOT COMPLETE	NOTES
1. Check the physician's order and institutional policy regarding PICC line blood draws.			
2. Check the orders for the lab work.			
3. Introduce yourself to the patient.			
4. Identify the patient by checking the wristband against the doctor's order and asking the patient, if conscious, to state his/her name.			
5. Verify the patient's allergy status.			
6. Explain the proposed procedure in terms the patient can understand.			
7. Gather all necessary equipment.			
8. Carry out proper hand hygiene.			
9. Provide for the patient's privacy.			
10. Set up equipment.			

(continues)

Skill 26 | *(continued)*

Name _____ Date _____ Instructor _____

ACTION TAKEN	COMPLETED SUCCESSFULLY	DID NOT COMPLETE	NOTES
11. Put on gloves.			
12. If an infusion is running, close the slide clamp. For 1 full minute prior to the blood draw, it is necessary to turn off all electrolyte and glucose-containing infusates that are infusing into other lumens.			
13. Instruct the patient to perform the Valsalva maneuver, during which time the administration set tubing is quickly disconnected from the pigtail, the pigtail is capped with the injection cap, and the distal end of the administration set is capped with the sterile cap.			
14. Prep the injection cap of the pigtail with the alcohol, followed by 2% CHG or iodophor.			
15. Attach a 10-ml saline-filled syringe. Open the slide clamp and ascertain placement and patency of the PICC, then vigorously flush with 10 ml of NS using the pulsatile, push-pause method. Clamp.			
16. Attach the vacuum container or the empty 10-ml or 20-ml syringe to the injection cap. Unclamp.			

Skill 26 | *(continued)*

Name _____ Date _____ Instructor _____

ACTION TAKEN	COMPLETED SUCCESSFULLY	DID NOT COMPLETE	NOTES
17. Draw 5 to 10 ml of blood into the discard tube.			
18. Quickly insert and fill the required blood-collection tube, then close the slide clamp on the pigtail and remove the vacuum container collecting device. Clamp.			
19. Prep the injection cap, open the slide clamp, and vigorously flush the line with at least 20 ml of NS to remove any residual blood. Clamp.			
20. Reconnect the infusion line and unclamp so the infusion may run (or unclamp, heparin-lock the pigtail, and then clamp).			
21. Dispose of used equipment and carry out proper hand hygiene.			
22. Document the procedure.			
23. Deliver the sample to the laboratory as soon as the blood draw is complete and integrity of the PICC is ensured.			

Skill 27 | PICC Exchange

Name _____ Date _____ Instructor _____

Approximate Time to Complete the Skill: 30 minutes

Overview of the Skill

A peripherally inserted central catheter (PICC) exchange is indicated when a catheter becomes irreversibly clotted or ruptured or is irreparable and the patient may not have another vein to support a PICC. It also is useful when a PICC is inadvertently partially pulled out. PICCs can be used for long-term infusion therapy. Some PICC lines have stayed in place for several months to years—all because of meticulous care and patients' compliance.

When an infection is suspected and the PICC must be removed to culture its tip, an exchange can be made to maintain the line while waiting for the results of the culture. An exchange also is a suitable procedure for conversion from a single-lumen to multi-lumen catheter and vice versa.

In most agencies, only registered nurses who are specially trained and certified by the employer are authorized to insert and exchange PICC lines. Preventing the need for catheter repair and exchange are major considerations for nurses. To maintain the integrity of the catheter, it is important to

- minimize catheter and catheter hub manipulations
- use 10 ml (or larger) capacity syringes to avoid over-pressurization of the catheter
- maintain dressings and tape to stabilize the catheter and any extensions.

If catheter repair is necessary, it is to be done with the appropriate repair kit, strictly following the manufacturer's guidelines. The nurse must never use a repair kit unless it is made by the manufacturer of the PICC being used. The nurse also must be specifically trained to perform PICC repairs.

ACTION TAKEN	COMPLETED SUCCESSFULLY	DID NOT COMPLETE	NOTES
1. Check the physician's order and institutional policy regarding PICC exchange.			
2. Introduce yourself to the patient.			
3. Identify the patient by checking the wristband against the doctor's order and asking the patient, if conscious, to state his/her name.			
4. Verify the patient's allergy status.			
5. Explain the proposed procedure in terms the patient can understand.			
6. Obtain the patient's consent for the procedure.			
7. Gather all necessary equipment.			

Skill 27 | (continued)

Name _____ Date _____ Instructor _____

ACTION TAKEN	COMPLETED SUCCESSFULLY	DID NOT COMPLETE	NOTES
8. Carry out proper hand hygiene.			
9. Provide privacy for the patient.			
10. Elevate the bed level.			
11. Secure all necessary supplies. The equipment and setup is the same as that for placing a new PICC, except for the use of an extra package of CHG or iodophor swabsticks.			
12. Place the patient comfortably in a semi-Fowler's position.			
13. Assess the patient's vital signs and level of consciousness. Record.			
14. Remove the PICC dressing.			
15. Following the procedure for inserting a new PICC, maintain a sterile field and drape the patient's arms appropriately.			
16. Don sterile gloves.			
17. Cover the end of the PICC with a sterile 4 × 4-inch gauze and remove the PICC from the insertion site to expose at least 5 inches of the line.			
18. Aseptically prepare the site, as for placement of a new PICC.			
19. Cleanse the existing PICC, using the additional CHG or iodophor swabsticks.			

 (continues)

Skill 27 | *(continued)*

Name _____ Date _____ Instructor _____

ACTION TAKEN	COMPLETED SUCCESSFULLY	DID NOT COMPLETE	NOTES
20. Clamp the PICC 1 inch distal to its exit site from the body.			
21. Cut the PICC 3 inches distal to the clamp. Discard the removed portion of the PICC off the sterile field.			
22. Remove the introducer needle from the plastic introducer sheath.			
23. Thread the plastic introducer sheath over the end of the exposed PICC and advance it up to the clamp.			
24. Fold the end of the PICC a short distance from the end of the introducer.			
25. While keeping the PICC doubled over, remove the clamp from its former position and place it between the introducer and the folded portion of the PICC.			
26. Advance the introducer sheath over the PICC up to its exit site on the arm.			
27. Apply normal saline around the PICC exit site and slowly advance the introducer into the site up to its hub.			
28. Gently pull down on the existing PICC.			
29. Pull the PICC out of the arm through the introducer.			

Skill 27 | *(continued)*

Name _____ Date _____ Instructor _____

ACTION TAKEN	COMPLETED SUCCESSFULLY	DID NOT COMPLETE	NOTES
Note: Following removal, there may be or may not be (more likely) a retrograde flow of blood from the introducer. To stimulate blood return, a tourniquet may be placed high on the upper arm. 30. Introduce the new PICC into the introducer and advance it to its premeasured insertion length, following the usual insertion protocols.			
31. Withdraw the introducer sheath and retract it from the PICC.			
32. Follow the same procedural guidelines for PICC placements, following advancement of the tip to its premeasured position.			
33. Lower the bed to standard low position, and raise the siderails.			
34. Remove personal protective equipment and dispose of used materials in appropriate waste containers.			
35. Carry out proper hand hygiene.			
36. Arrange for portable chest x-ray or transfer to radiology for x-ray.			
37. Document the procedure.			

Skill 28 | PICC Removal

Name _____ Date _____ Instructor _____

Approximate Time to Complete the Skill: 5–10 minutes

Overview of the Skill

Once a peripherallyi inserted central catheter (PICC) is no longer needed, it should be removed. Sometimes, even though it is still needed, the PICC must be removed (usually because of infection or the client's inability to comply with the protocols for keeping it in place).

ACTION TAKEN	COMPLETED SUCCESSFULLY	DID NOT COMPLETE	NOTES
1. Check the physician's order and institutional policy regarding PICC removal.			
2. Introduce yourself to the patient.			
3. Identify the patient by checking the wristband against the doctor's order and asking the patient, if conscious, to state his/her name.			
4. Verify the patient's allergy status.			
5. Explain the proposed procedure in terms the patient can understand.			
6. Obtain the patient's consent for the procedure.			
7. Gather all necessary equipment.			
8. Carry out proper hand hygiene.			
9. Provide for the patient's privacy.			
10. Elevate the bed level.			
11. Secure all necessary supplies.			
12. Position the patient comfortably in a supine or semi-Fowler's position with the arm extended at a 45- to 90-degree angle from the torso.			
13. Flush the PICC with normal saline.			

Skill 28 | *(continued)*

Name _____ Date _____ Instructor _____

ACTION TAKEN	COMPLETED SUCCESSFULLY	DID NOT COMPLETE	NOTES
14. Don disposable gloves.			
15. Remove the dressing (and sutures, if present).			
16. If a culture is required, cleanse the PICC exit site.			
17. Gently grasp the catheter at its exit site from the skin.			
18. Remove the catheter, pulling it straight out while maintaining gentle, constant traction and regrasping the catheter every few centimeters.			
19. Measure the length of the removed catheter and compare it to the documented length that was inserted.			
20. Gently apply pressure with the 4 × 4-inch gauze.			
21. Fold the gauze over and apply a strip of tape or an adhesive bandage. Leave the dressing in place for 24 hours.			
22. Discard the catheter into the sharps container.			
23. Lower the bed to standard low position, and raise siderails.			
24. Remove personal protective equipment and dispose of it in the appropriate container.			
25. Carry out proper hand hygiene.			
26. Document the procedure.			

Skill 29 | Preparation of the VAP Access Site

Name _____ Date _____ Instructor _____

Approximate Time to Complete the Skill: 5 minutes

Overview of the Skill

Before accessing a vascular access port (VAP), the site should be inspected and prepared. To prepare the VAP site for use requires cleansing the insertion area aseptically.

ACTION TAKEN	COMPLETED SUCCESSFULLY	DID NOT COMPLETE	NOTES
1. Check the physician's order and institutional policy regarding VAP access.			
2. Introduce yourself to the patient.			
3. Identify the patient by checking the wristband against the doctor's order and asking the patient, if conscious, to state his/her name.			
4. Verify the patient's allergy status.			
5. Explain the proposed procedure in terms the patient can understand.			
6. Obtain the patient's consent for the procedure.			
7. Gather all necessary equipment.			
8. Carry out proper hand hygiene.			
9. Provide for the patient's privacy.			
10. Elevate the bed level.			
11. Secure all necessary supplies.			
12. Inspect the site.			
13. Wash the insertion area with soap, rinse well with water, and pat dry.			

Skill 29 | *(continued)*

Name _____ Date _____ Instructor _____

ACTION TAKEN	COMPLETED SUCCESSFULLY	DID NOT COMPLETE	NOTES
14. Review the Valsalva maneuver with the patient.			
15. Assess vital signs and level of consciousness, and record.			
16. Set up the equipment in a sterile manner.			
17. Expose the skin and palpate for the septum.			
18. Don gown, mask, and sterile gloves.			
19. Instruct the patient to turn his/her head away from the VAP site.			
20. Cleanse the septum site with a 70% isopropyl alcohol swabstick, starting at the intended puncture site and moving outward in a concentric circle 4 to 5 inches in diameter. Repeat for a total of three times, using a different swabstick each time. Allow the area to air-dry.			
21. Repeat the above steps, using the 2% CHG or iodophor swabsticks, and allow the area to air-dry after the third application.			
22. Gently wipe off any residue of the iodophor at the needle-insertion site.			

Skill 30 | Accessing and Deaccessing the VAP

Name _____ Date _____ Instructor _____

Approximate Time to Complete the Skill: 10 minutes for accessing and 5 minutes for deaccessing

Overview of the Skill

Note: This skill covers access and deaccess of single and double vascular access ports (VAPs). To administer a bolus injection and deliver an infusion into a vascular access port, review the procedure in Skills 31 and 32 for bolus injection and continuous infusion via a VAP.

A subcutaneous vascular access device (VAD) is an implantable port, sometimes called a vascular access port (VAP). It functions in much the same manner as a central venous catheter (CVC) but is inserted surgically in a subcutaneous area under the skin without any portion exiting the body. The ports are not externally exposed, so they are cosmetically appealing, the risk of infection is reduced, and patients can carry out virtually all activities without the need for care of the exit site more frequently than every 4–6 weeks, or routine heparin or saline flushing if the ports are not being used.

The VAP sits in a surgically incised subcutaneous pocket located centrally or peripherally. The design allows for repeated entry into the vascular system, through percutaneous needle insertions, to deliver IV fluids, medications, blood or blood products, chemotherapy, and total parenteral nutrition, and to withdraw blood samples. Implantable ports are indicated for patients who require vascular access for long-term infusion therapy but usually do not receive infusions or have blood samples drawn more frequently than every 1–3 weeks. VAPs are indicated for all of the same reasons as tunneled and nontunneled CVCs.

The catheter of a VAP may be an open-ended system or a closed system (Groshong®). When used to deliver chemotherapy or other medications, the catheter tip also may be placed in various body cavities such as the epidural space, the pleural cavity, and the peritoneum, as well as the arteries or vessels that lead into major organs such as the liver or pancreas.

The top of the VAP consists of a domed, single or double injection port with a self-sealing silicone septum (partition) that is connected to a radiopaque catheter, the distal portion of which is positioned in the superior vena cava. The domed portion can be accessed repeatedly with a noncoring, nonbarbed needle. Because the VAP is not visible from the skin surface, it must be palpated to be accessed.

Regular hypodermic needles, because of their design, can damage the portal septum. Noncoring needles have a deflected point that helps avoid septal injury. The type of noncoring, nonbarbed needle used most commonly is the Huber™ Needle. It is available with or without Luer-Lok® extension tubings (Y-site or non-Y-site) and either is straight or has a right-angle configuration. The right-angled needles are recommended for continuous or intermittent infusions, because of their low profile and ease of securing. These needles may be left in place for up to 7 days, at which time they must be changed if continued infusions are indicated. The straight needles generally are used only for bolus injections or blood sampling.

ACTION TAKEN	COMPLETED SUCCESSFULLY	DID NOT COMPLETE	NOTES
1. Check the physician's order and institutional policy regarding VAP access.			
2. Introduce yourself to the patient.			
3. Identify the patient by checking the wristband against the doctor's order and asking the patient, if conscious, to state his/her name.			

Skill 30 | *(continued)*

Name _____ Date _____ Instructor _____

ACTION TAKEN	COMPLETED SUCCESSFULLY	DID NOT COMPLETE	NOTES
4. Verify the patient's allergy status.			
5. Explain the proposed procedure in terms the patient can understand.			
6. Obtain the patient's consent for the procedure.			
7. Gather all necessary equipment.			
8. Carry out proper hand hygiene.			
9–22. Prepare the site as outlined in Skill 29, steps 9–22.			
For Single Port Access:			
23. Administer local anesthesia, if indicated, following agency protocols.			
24. Connect the needle with extension set to the 10-ml syringe filled with NS, and clear the tubing of air, taking care not to contaminate the equipment, the site, or the nurse's gloved hands.			
25. Locate the base of the port with the nondominant hand. Triangulate the port between the thumb and the first two fingers of the nondominant hand. Approximate the center of the port and aim for the center of these three fingers.			
26. Instruct the patient to perform the Valsalva maneuver.			

(continues)

Skill 30 | (continued)

Name _____ Date _____ Instructor _____

ACTION TAKEN	COMPLETED SUCCESSFULLY	DID NOT COMPLETE	NOTES
27. Insert the needle perpendicular to the port septum. Advance the needle through the skin and septum until reaching the bottom of the reservoir. Instruct the patient to breathe normally.			
28. Aspirate for a blood return. Do not inject until placement is confirmed.			
29. Flush the line vigorously, using the push-pause, pulsatile method.			
30. Continue with the procedure for administering the bolus injection, continuous/ intermittent infusion, flushing, and heparin-locking, as indicated.			
For Dual Port Access:			
1–22. Prepare the site as outlined in Skill 29, steps 9–22.			
23. Administer local anesthesia, if indicated, following agency protocols.			
24. Connect the needle with extension set to the 10-ml syringe filled with NS, and clear the tubing of air, taking care not to con-taminate the equipment, the site, or the nurse's gloved hands.			

Skill 30 | *(continued)*

Name _____ Date _____ Instructor _____

ACTION TAKEN	COMPLETED SUCCESSFULLY	DID NOT COMPLETE	NOTES
25. Palpate to locate the port septum to be accessed. a. With the nondominant hand, locate the base of the port. b. Approximate the center of the dual port and place the index finger of the dominant hand to mark the spot. c. Triangulate the right or left side of the dual port between the thumb and first two fingers of the dominant hand. Aim for the center point of these three fingers.			
26. Instruct the patient to perform the Valsalva maneuver.			
27. Insert the needle perpendicular to the port septum. Advance the needle through the skin and septum until reaching the bottom of the reservoir. Instruct the patient to breathe normally.			
28. Aspirate for a blood return. Do not inject until placement is confirmed.			
29. Flush the line vigorously, using the push-pause, pulsatile method.			

(continues)

Skill 30 | *(continued)*

Name _____ Date _____ Instructor _____

ACTION TAKEN	COMPLETED SUCCESSFULLY	DID NOT COMPLETE	NOTES
30. Access each septum separately, and flush with normal saline.			
31. Continue with the procedure for administering the bolus injection, continuous/ intermittent infusion, flushing, and heparin-locking, as indicated.			
To Deaccess the VAP:			
32. Prior to with-drawing the needle, stabilize the port with two fingers.			
33. Instruct the patient to perform the Valsalva maneuver.			
34. Slowly remove a noncoring needle while injecting the last 0.5 ml of infusate. Instruct the patient to breathe normally.			
35. Dispose of used equipment and carry out proper hand hygiene.			
36. Document the procedure.			

Skill 31 | Bolus Injection via the VAP

Name _____ Date _____ Instructor _____

Approximate Time to Complete the Skill: 15 minutes

Overview of the Skill

Note: This skill covers bolus injection into a vascular access port (VAP). Before examining this skill, you must have completed the procedure covering the access and deaccess of single and double vascular access ports. Please review Skill 30, "Accessing and Deaccessing the VAP."

Implantable ports are indicated for patients who require vascular access for long-term infusion therapy but usually do not receive infusions or have blood samples drawn more frequently than every 1–3 weeks. They are indicated for all of the same reasons as tunneled and nontunneled CVCs.

The top of the VAP consists of a domed, single or double injection port with a self-sealing silicone septum (partition) that is connected to a radiopaque catheter, the distal portion of which is positioned in the superior vena cava. The domed portion can be accessed repeatedly with a noncoring, nonbarbed needle. Because the VAP is not visible from the skin surface, it must be palpated to be accessed.

Regular hypodermic needles, because of their design, can damage the portal septum. Noncoring needles have a deflected point that helps avoid septal injury. The type of noncoring, nonbarbed needle used most commonly is the Huber™ needle. It is available with or without Luer-Lok® extension tubings (Y-site or non-Y-site), and either is straight or has a right-angle configuration. The right-angled needles are recommended for continuous or intermittent infusions because of their low profile and ease of securing. The needles may be left in place for up to 7 days, at which time they must be changed if continued infusions are indicated. The straight needles generally are used only for bolus injections or blood sampling.

ACTION TAKEN	COMPLETED SUCCESSFULLY	DID NOT COMPLETE	NOTES
1. Check the physician's order and institutional policy regarding VAP access.			
2. Introduce yourself to the patient.			
3. Identify the patient by checking the wristband against the doctor's order and asking the patient, if conscious, to state his/her name.			
4. Verify the patient's allergy status.			
5. Explain the proposed procedure in terms the patient can understand.			
6. Gather all necessary equipment.			
7. Carry out proper hand hygiene.			
8. Provide privacy.			
9. Elevate the bed level.			

(continues)

Skill 31 | *(continued)*

Name _____ Date _____ Instructor _____

ACTION TAKEN	COMPLETED SUCCESSFULLY	DID NOT COMPLETE	NOTES
10. Secure all necessary supplies.			
11. Inspect the site.			
12. Wash the insertion area with soap, rinse well with water, and pat dry.			
13. Review the Valsalva maneuver with the patient.			
14. Assess vital signs and level of consciousness. Record.			
15. Set up the equipment in a sterile manner.			
16. Expose the skin, and palpate for the septum.			
17. Don gown, mask, and sterile gloves.			
18. Instruct the patient to turn his/her head away from the VAP site.			
19. Cleanse the septum site with a 70% isopropyl alcohol swabstick, starting at the intended puncture site and moving outward in a concentric circle 4 to 5 inches in diameter. Repeat for a total of three times, using a different swabstick each time. Allow the area to air-dry.			
20. Repeat the preceding steps, using the 2% CHG or iodophor swabsticks. After the third application, allow the area to air-dry.			

Skill 31 | *(continued)*

Name _____ Date _____ Instructor _____

ACTION TAKEN	COMPLETED SUCCESSFULLY	DID NOT COMPLETE	NOTES
21. Gently wipe off any residue of the iodophor at the needle-insertion site.			
22. Administer local anesthesia, if indicated, following agency protocols.			
23. Connect the appropriate needle with extension set to the 10-ml syringe filled with NS, and prime the tubing and needle to displace any air, taking care not to contaminate the equipment, the site, or your gloved hands.			
24. Triangulate the port between the thumb and the first two fingers of the non-dominant hand. Aim for the center point of these three fingers.			
25. Instruct the patient to perform the Valsalva maneuver.			
26. Insert the needle perpendicular to the port septum. Advance the needle through the skin and septum until it reaches the bottom of the reservoir. Instruct the patient to breathe normally.			
27. Aspirate for a blood return. Do not inject until placement is confirmed.			
28. Vigorously flush the line, using the push-pause, pulsatile method.			

(continues)

Skill 31 | *(continued)*

Name _____ Date _____ Instructor _____

ACTION TAKEN	COMPLETED SUCCESSFULLY	DID NOT COMPLETE	NOTES
29. Close the slide clamp on the extension tubing as the last 0.5 ml of NS is injected.			
30. Instruct the patient to perform the Valsalva maneuver.			
31. Disconnect the empty NS saline syringe and attach the 10-ml syringe containing the bolus medication. Instruct the patient to breathe normally.			
32. Open the slide clamp on the extension tubing and administer the drug, according to directions, while examining the injection site.			
33. When the injection is complete, clamp the extension set.			
34. Instruct the patient to perform the Valsalva maneuver. Remove the syringe.			
35. Attach the 10-ml syringe containing the NS. Instruct the patient to breathe normally.			
36. Open the slide clamp on the extension tubing, and flush the line vigorously, using the pulsatile, push-pause method.			
37. Clamp the line as the last 0.5 ml is instilled.			

Skill 31 | *(continued)*

Name _____ Date _____ Instructor _____

ACTION TAKEN	COMPLETED SUCCESSFULLY	DID NOT COMPLETE	NOTES
38. Instruct the patient to perform the Valsalva maneuver. Detach the empty NS syringe. If the VAP has a Groshong® tip, remove the needle at this time, and do not flush with heparin.			
39. Attach the 10-ml syringe containing the heparin flush.			
40. Instruct the patient to breathe normally. Open the slide clamp on the extension tubing.			
41. Heparin-lock the port, closing the slide clamp as the last 0.5 ml is injected.			
42. Stabilize the port with two fingers, instruct the patient to perform the Valsalva maneuver, and remove the needle. Instruct the patient to breathe normally.			
43. Return the bed to the low position and raise the siderails.			
44. Dispose of used equipment, and carry out proper hand hygiene.			
45. Document the procedure.			

Skill 32 | Continuous Infusion via the VAP

Name _____ Date _____ Instructor _____

Approximate Time to Complete the Skill: 15 minutes

Overview of the Skill

Note: This skill covers continuous infusion into a vascular access port (VAP). Before examining this skill, you must have completed the procedure covering the access and deaccess of single and double vascular access ports. Please review Skill 30, "Accessing and Deaccessing the VAP."

Implantable ports are indicated for patients who require vascular access for long-term infusion therapy but usually do not receive infusions or have blood samples drawn more frequently than every 1–3 weeks. These are indicated for all of the same reasons as tunneled and nontunneled CVCs.

The top of the VAP consists of a domed, single or double injection port with a self-sealing silicone septum (partition) that is connected to a radiopaque catheter, the distal portion of which is positioned in the superior vena cava. The domed portion can be accessed repeatedly with a noncoring, nonbarbed needle. Because the VAP is not visible from the skin surface, it must be palpated to be accessed.

Regular hypodermic needles, because of their design, can damage the portal septum. Noncoring needles have a deflected point that helps avoid septal injury. The most commonly used type of noncoring, nonbarbed needle is the Huber™ needle.

It is available with or without Luer-Lok® extension tubings (Y-site or non-Y-site), and either is straight or has a right-angle configuration. The right-angled needles are recommended for continuous or intermittent infusions, because of their low profile and ease of securing. The needles may be left in place for up to 7 days, at which time they must be changed if continued infusions are indicated. The straight needles generally are used only for bolus injections or blood sampling.

ACTION TAKEN	COMPLETED SUCCESSFULLY	DID NOT COMPLETE	NOTES
1. Check the physician's order.			
2. Introduce yourself to the patient.			
3. Identify the patient by checking the wristband against the doctor's order and asking the patient, if conscious, to state his/her name.			
4. Verify the patient's allergy status.			
5. Explain the proposed procedure in terms the patient can understand.			
6. Gather all necessary equipment.			
7. Carry out proper hand hygiene.			
8. Provide for the patient's privacy.			
9. Elevate the bed level.			

Skill 32 | *(continued)*

Name _____ Date _____ Instructor _____

ACTION TAKEN	COMPLETED SUCCESSFULLY	DID NOT COMPLETE	NOTES
10. Secure all necessary supplies.			
11. Inspect the site.			
12. Wash the insertion area with soap, rinse well with water, and pat dry.			
13. Review the Valsalva maneuver with the patient.			
14. Assess vital signs and level of consciousness. Record.			
15. Set up the equipment in a sterile manner.			
16. Expose the skin, and palpate for the septum.			
17. Don gown, mask, and sterile gloves.			
18. Instruct the patient to turn his/her head away from the VAP site.			
19. Cleanse the septum site with a 70% isopropyl alcohol swabstick, starting at the intended puncture site and moving outward in a concentric circle 4 to 5 inches in diameter. Repeat for a total of three times, using a different swabstick each time. Allow the area to air-dry.			
20. Repeat the preceding steps, using the 2% CHG or iodophor swabsticks. After the third application, allow the area to air-dry.			

(continues)

Skill 32 | *(continued)*

Name _____ Date _____ Instructor _____

ACTION TAKEN	COMPLETED SUCCESSFULLY	DID NOT COMPLETE	NOTES
21. Gently wipe off any residue of the iodophor at the needle-insertion site.			
22. Administer local anesthesia, if indicated, following agency protocol.			
23. Connect the appropriate needle with extension set to the 10-ml syringe filled with NS. Prime the tubing and needle to displace any air, taking care not to contaminate the equipment, the site, or your gloved hands.			
24. Triangulate the port between the thumb and the first two fingers of the non-dominant hand. Aim for the center point of these three fingers.			
25. Instruct the patient to perform the Valsalva maneuver.			
26. Insert the needle perpendicular to the port septum. Advance the needle through the skin and septum until it reaches the bottom of the reservoir. Instruct the patient to breathe normally.			
27. Aspirate for a blood return. Do not inject until placement is confirmed.			
28. Flush the line vigorously, using the push-pause, pulsatile method.			

Skill 32 | *(continued)*

Name _____ Date _____ Instructor _____

ACTION TAKEN	COMPLETED SUCCESSFULLY	DID NOT COMPLETE	NOTES
29. Close the slide clamp on the extension tubing as the last 0.5 ml of NS is injected.			
30. Place the 2 × 2-inch gauze (rolled up or folded in 4s) under the needle hub. Secure the needle and dressing in place with the transparent dressing.			
31. Open the slide clamp and flush the line vigorously, using the pulsatile, push-pause method.			
32. Clamp the line. Instruct the patient to perform the Valsalva maneuver. Disconnect the syringe.			
33. Connect the fluid delivery system. Instruct the patient to breathe normally.			
34. If an electronic infusion device is used, turn it on, open the slide clamp, and initiate the infusion.			
35. Examine the site for signs of extravasation, and initiate the appropriate interventions if needed.			
36. Tape all tubing connections with the paper tape.			

(continues)

Skill 32 | *(continued)*

Name _____ Date _____ Instructor _____

ACTION TAKEN	COMPLETED SUCCESSFULLY	DID NOT COMPLETE	NOTES
37. When the infusion is complete, turn off the electronic infusion device (EID), clamp the extension set, and instruct the patient to perform the Valsalva maneuver. Disconnect the IV line from the extension tubing of the needle.			
38. Connect the 20-ml syringe containing the NS. Have the patient breathe normally. Open the slide clamp and flush vigorously, as before.			
39. Heparin-lock the port (unless it has a Groshong® tip), closing the slide clamp as the last 0.5 ml is injected.			
40. Stabilize the port with two fingers, and instruct the patient to perform the Valsalva maneuver. Remove the needle, and instruct the patient to breathe normally.			
41. Return the bed to the low position and raise the siderails.			
42. Dispose of used equipment and carry out proper hand hygiene.			
43. Document the procedure.			

Skill 33 | Blood Sampling from the VAP

Name _____ Date _____ Instructor _____

Approximate Time to Complete the Skill: 10 minutes

Overview of the Skill

Patients who have an implantable vascular access port (VAP) may have blood drawn from the port. Because it eliminates the need for repeated venipuncture, it makes the patient more comfortable and reduces the risk for injury.

Some sources state that certain blood tests should not be run on samples taken from an IV that has been used to infuse certain medications. Peak and trough levels for antibiotics may be more accurate if drawn peripherally rather than from the central line used for administration. This may not be possible for a patient who has poor peripheral access.

In most agencies, only registered nurses who are trained to work with central lines and care for patients who have them are authorized to draw blood specimens from VAPs. An ALERT sign, stating that RNs only are to draw blood, is placed over the head of the patient's bed and on the chart to prevent needless attempts at peripheral blood sampling.

ACTION TAKEN	COMPLETED SUCCESSFULLY	DID NOT COMPLETE	NOTES
1. Check the physician's order.			
2. Check the orders for lab work.			
3. Introduce yourself to the patient.			
4. Identify the patient by checking the wristband against the doctor's order and asking the patient, if conscious, to state his/her name.			
5. Verify the patient's allergy status.			
6. Explain the proposed procedure in terms the patient can understand.			
7. Gather all necessary equipment. Prior to beginning the procedure, have all necessary heparin and saline drawn up.			
8. Carry out proper hand hygiene.			
9. Provide for the patient's privacy.			
10. Set up equipment.			
11. Put on gloves.			

(continues)

Skill 33 | (continued)

Name _____ Date _____ Instructor _____

ACTION TAKEN	COMPLETED SUCCESSFULLY	DID NOT COMPLETE	NOTES
12. Aseptically prepare the injection site (following the procedure for accessing and deaccessing the VAP, Skill 30).			
13. Flush the extension tubing, stopcock, and needle, maintaining sterility.			
14. Insert the needle, aspirate for a blood return, and flush the port vigorously with 5 ml of NS.			
15. Withdraw at least 5 ml of blood, and discard the syringe into the sharps container.			
16. Aspirate the desired blood volume into the 20-ml syringe and transfer it to the appropriate blood sample tube (or use a Vacutainer® per the manufacturer's protocol).			
17. Flush the system vigorously with 20 ml of sterile NS, using the push-pause, pulsatile method.			
18. Heparin-lock the system (for ports with open-ended catheters).			
19. Label the blood tubes, and deliver the sample to the laboratory as soon as the blood draw is complete and integrity of the VAP is ensured.			
20. Dispose of used equipment and carry out proper hand hygiene.			
21. Document the procedure.			

Skill 34 | Clearing a Blocked VAP

Name _____ Date _____ Instructor _____

Approximate Time to Complete the Skill: 15–20 minutes plus time for declotting agent to work

Overview of the Skill

Note: Prior to reading this, review Skill 30, "Accessing and Deaccessing the VAP." The principles involved are the same as for clearing occlusions in any central venous catheter (CVC). The method of access, however, is different.

VAPs can become occluded for various reasons. Withdrawal (or aspiration) occlusion (which is not a true occlusion because the infusion passage is not obstructed) is usually the result of the formation of a fibrin sheath or fibrin tail, or because the opening of the catheter tip lumen is pressed against the wall of the vessel. The latter situation usually can be alleviated by repositioning the patient or having the patient perform the Valsalva maneuver.

Possible causes of true catheter occlusion include

- improper flushing or irrigation (failure to use pulsatile, push-pause flushing)
- clot formation at the lumen exit
- obstruction by drug precipitates
- obstruction by lipid deposition
- catheter displacement
- restriction of catheter flow by sutures that have tightened around the circumference of the catheter
- coiling, kinking, or pinching of the catheter between the clavicle and the first rib
- catheter damage or transection from repeated pressure of the clavicle and the first rib on the catheter during normal movement if it is placed through the "pinch-off" area.

Treatment of any occlusion involves eliminating the cause. The nurse may aspirate a blood clot or dissolve it. The procedures for clearing catheters occluded by clots, lipids, and some precipitates are presented below.

Clearing a Blocked Catheter

Resolution of precipitate occlusions is based on the principle of returning the precipitate into solution by altering the pH of the material causing the occlusion.

For dosage accuracy, use a tuberculin syringe to draw up the medication. The volume of the agent instilled should be approximately equal to the volume of the catheter so the agent remains in the catheter and is not advanced into the bloodstream.

For clots, use

- normal saline (NS) (5 ml) for the POP method
- Activase® (tissue plasminogen activator [TPA]) from the pharmacy, already reconstituted to a dilution of 1 mg/I ml.

For lipid deposits, use

- ethanol 70% (1 ml), following the procedure for Activase® instillation.

For decreased pH (acid residues, minerals such as calcium phosphate, precipitates, and most antibiotics), use

- hydrochloric acid 0.1 N/ml (1 ml), following the procedure for Activase® instillation.

For increased pH (alkaline residues), use

- sodium bicarbonate 1 mEq/ml (1 ml), following the procedure for Activase® instillation.

(continues)

Skill 34 | *(continued)*

Name _____ Date _____ Instructor _____

ACTION TAKEN	COMPLETED SUCCESSFULLY	DID NOT COMPLETE	NOTES
1. Check the physician's order.			
2. Introduce yourself to the patient.			
3. Identify the patient by checking the wristband against the doctor's order and asking the patient, if conscious, to state his/her name.			
4. Verify the patient's allergy status.			
5. Explain the proposed procedure in terms the patient can understand.			
6. Gather all necessary equipment.			
7. Carry out proper hand hygiene.			
8. Access the port.			
9. Using the 35-ml syringe, gently instill the declotting agent. Use a gentle pull-push action on the syringe to maximize mixing of the solution within the port and catheter.			
10. Leave the declotting agent in place for 15 minutes.			
11. Attempt to aspirate the declotting solution and the clot.			
12. Once the blockage has been cleared, flush the catheter vigorously with at least 10 ml of NS, using the pulsatile, push-pause method.			
13. Heparin-lock the port (for open-ended catheters).			

Skill 34 | *(continued)*

Name _____ Date _____ Instructor _____

Alternative (Two-Needle) Declotting Method

An alternative method for declotting a VAP involves the use of two noncoring access needles. This method is especially useful when the blockage is in the port itself. Although it can be done by one nurse, it is accomplished more easily by two nurses (with one maneuvering the syringe containing the declotting agent and the other pulling back on the empty syringe).

ACTION TAKEN	COMPLETED SUCCESSFULLY	DID NOT COMPLETE	NOTES
1. Check the physician's order.			
2. Introduce yourself to the patient.			
3. Identify the patient by checking the wristband against the doctor's order and asking the patient, if conscious, to state his/her name.			
4. Verify the patient's allergy status.			
5. Explain the proposed procedure in terms the patient can understand.			
6. Carry out proper hand hygiene.			
7. Connect the extension sets to each needle and syringe. Purge the air from the extension set and needle connected to the syringe containing the declotting agent.			
8. Access the port with both needles.			
9. Using the empty syringe, try the POP method to dislodge the clot. If this doesn't work, proceed to step 10.			

(continues)

Skill 34 | *(continued)*

Name _____ Date _____ Instructor _____

ACTION TAKEN	COMPLETED SUCCESSFULLY	DID NOT COMPLETE	NOTES
10. Gently instill a small volume of the declotting agent into the port, then pull back on the plunger of the empty syringe. Continue to push and pull gently until all the declotting agent has been instilled.			
11. Once the blockage has been cleared, flush the catheter vigorously with at least 10 ml of NS, using the pulsatile, push-pause method.			
12. Heparin-lock the port (for open-ended catheters).			

If the preceding methods do not remove the clot or obstruction, the blockage may be farther down in the catheter. When this seems to be the problem, it is advisable to try the negative pressure method of declotting, using a stopcock. (See Skill 20, "The Stopcock-Negative Pressure Method.")

Skill 35 | Accessing and Deaccessing the CathLink™ 20 Implanted Port

Name _____ Date _____ Instructor _____

Approximate Time to Complete the Skill: 10 minutes

Overview of the Skill

The CathLink™ 20 is connected to an open-ended catheter. Access is obtained by percutaneous insertions of a 20-gauge, over-the-needle IV catheter (ONC), with a minimum length of 1¾ inches. The funnel-shaped entrance to the port guides the ONC into the angled access pathway. The layered septum seals around the flexible catheter tip once it has been advanced and the needle has been removed. Noncoring needles should not be used with this type of port.

ACTION TAKEN	COMPLETED SUCCESSFULLY	DID NOT COMPLETE	NOTES
1. Check the physician's order.			
2. Introduce yourself to the patient.			
3. Identify the patient by checking the wristband against the doctor's order and asking the patient, if conscious, to state his/her name.			
4. Verify the patient's allergy status, and assess for allergies, especially to iodine.			
5. Explain the proposed procedure in terms the patient can understand.			
6. Gather all necessary equipment.			
7. Carry out proper hand hygiene.			
8. Provide for the patient's privacy.			
9. Elevate the bed level.			
10. Secure all necessary supplies.			
11. Inspect the site.			
12. Wash the insertion area with soap, rinse well with water, and pat dry.			
13. Review the Valsalva maneuver with the patient.			

(continues)

Skill 35 | (continued)

Name _____ Date _____ Instructor _____

ACTION TAKEN	COMPLETED SUCCESSFULLY	DID NOT COMPLETE	NOTES
14. Assess vital signs and level of consciousness. Record.			
15. Set up the equipment in a sterile manner.			
16. Cleanse the septum site with a 70% isopropyl alcohol swabstick, starting at the intended puncture site and moving outward in a concentric circle 4 to 5 inches in diameter. Repeat for a total of three times, using a fresh swabstick each time. Allow the area to air-dry.			
17. Repeat the preceding steps, using the 2% CHG or iodophor swabsticks. After the third application, allow the area to air-dry.			
18. Attach to the extension set a 10-ml syringe filled with sterile NS. Expel air and close the clamp.			
19. Using a sterile gloved hand, locate the CathLink™ 20 implanted port and palpate to identify the funnel-shaped entrance.			
20. Stabilize the port by holding it between the thumb and forefinger of the nondominant hand.			

Skill 35 | *(continued)*

Name _____ Date _____ Instructor _____

ACTION TAKEN	COMPLETED SUCCESSFULLY	DID NOT COMPLETE	NOTES
21. Aim for the funnel-shaped entrance (between two fingers), and insert the ONC into the port's funnel-shaped entrance until resistance is felt.			
22. Ask the patient to perform the Valsalva maneuver.			
23. Using the thumb and forefinger of the dominant hand, advance the ONC completely into the port by grasping and advancing the catheter hub only, while simultaneously withdrawing the needle. (This also can be accomplished by advancing the ONC with one hand and withdrawing the needle with the other hand.) The IV catheter should be advanced a minimum of 1 cm.			
24. Place a gloved finger over the IV catheter hub until a secondary device can be attached.			
25. Immediately attach the syringe or extension set to the ONC. Instruct the patient to breathe normally.			
26. Dispose of the needle/stylet in the sharps container.			
27. Aspirate for a blood return.			
28. Flush with NS.			
29. Proceed with the infusion protocol.			

(continues)

Skill 35 | *(continued)*

Name _____ Date _____ Instructor _____

ACTION TAKEN	COMPLETED SUCCESSFULLY	DID NOT COMPLETE	NOTES
30. Following injection of medication/ infusion, flush the port with normal saline.			
31. Heparin-lock the port.			
32. To deaccess the port, stabilize the CathLink™ 20 with two fingers.			
33. Remove the ONC slowly while injecting the last 0.5 ml of infusate.			
34. Return the bed to the low position and raise the siderails.			
35. Dispose of used equipment and carry out proper hand hygiene.			
36. Document the procedure.			

Skill 36 | Transfusion of Blood Components

Name _____ Date _____ Instructor _____

Approximate Time to Complete the Skill: 15 minutes to initiate the infusion, 30 minutes to 2 hours to monitor the patient during the infusion, and 10 minutes to discontinue the infusion and complete the documentation

Overview of the Skill

The blood and its components are life-sustaining constituents. Transfusion therapy is a major multidisciplinary health-care responsibility with a myriad of significant implications. The registered professional nurse is responsible for administering and monitoring the transfusion of these products, based on the physician's order and the patient's condition. A high level of knowledge and skill is fundamental to proper administration and management.

Before a transfusion can be administered, the donor's blood type and the recipient's blood type have to be ascertained and correctly matched for compatibility. This process is referred to as blood typing and crossmatching (T & C). Minor crossmatching tests for compatibility are done by mixing the donor's serum and the recipient's blood. Major crossmatching consists of mixing the donor's red blood cells (RBCs) and the recipient's serum. Prior to administering the transfusion, blood is typed, crossmatched, and stored in a blood bank or a blood-processing service.

It is extremely important for everyone to know his/her blood type, in case the need for surgery or an emergency arises and necessitates a transfusion. If the blood of a donor and recipient are incompatible, agglutination obstructs blood vessels, which in turn prevents circulatory flow and precipitates death.

Administration of Transfusion

In accordance with the regulations set forth by governmental agencies, the American Association of Blood Banks, the Intravenous Nurses Society, and the policies and procedures set forth by the employer, as well as the Nurse Practice Act of the state in which the nurse is licensed, the registered professional nurse is responsible for the patient's safety during all aspects of blood transfusion therapy. The nurse is expected to continually assess, evaluate, and document the patient's responses in the period preceding administration, throughout the transfusion, as it is discontinued, and during the post-transfusion period. The nurse must have knowledge and understanding of immunohematology, blood grouping, blood and blood components, administration equipment and the techniques appropriate for each component, and transfusion reactions, as well as the potential risks to the patient and the nurse. Blood or its constituents can be administered only with medical authorization and proper consent.

ACTION TAKEN	COMPLETED SUCCESSFULLY	DID NOT COMPLETE	NOTES
1. Verify the prescriber's order.			
2. Verify informed consent. a. Assess the patient's understanding of the procedure, then describe the procedure and provide the patient with the opportunity to ask questions and vent concerns.			

(continues)

Skill 36 | *(continued)*

Name _____ Date _____ Instructor _____

ACTION TAKEN	COMPLETED SUCCESSFULLY	DID NOT COMPLETE	NOTES
b. Ask if he/she has ever had any type of transfusion in the past (including cryoprecipitate, FFP, platelets, and RBCs). c. During the transfusion, assess for a reaction any symptoms that may be misinterpreted. If possible—although not absolutely contraindicated—transfusion should be avoided in febrile (fever >38°C or 100.4°F) patients.			
3. Verify the patient's identity. If he/she is conscious, ask the patient to state his/her full name. The patient must have an identification band as well as a blood administration I.D. bracelet (put on by the blood administration service when a blood sample was drawn for typing and crossmatching). Validate that the name and numbers on both I.D. bands correlate with those on the patient's chart and on the laboratory forms for pretransfusion testing of the blood.			

Skill 36 | *(continued)*

Name _____ Date _____ Instructor _____

ACTION TAKEN	COMPLETED SUCCESSFULLY	DID NOT COMPLETE	NOTES
4. If the patient is ambulatory, it is recommend that he/she go to the bathroom and empty the bladder. If bedridden, provide a bedpan (for females) or urinal (for males).			
5. Assemble all necessary equipment and start an infusion of 0.9% NaCl, if ordered, using the appropriate administration set, filter, and proper cannula size. Never piggyback blood into an existing IV line. Obtain an extra set of tubing and a container of 0.9% NaCl (neither of which is opened, or charged to the patient) and leave them at the bedside. Locate the availability of emergency drugs.			
6. Premedicate the patient with antihistamines, antipyretics, or diuretics, as ordered by the physician.			

(continues)

Skill 36 | *(continued)*

Name _____ Date _____ Instructor _____

ACTION TAKEN	COMPLETED SUCCESSFULLY	DID NOT COMPLETE	NOTES
7. Just prior to its administration, obtain the blood component from the transfusion service. Unless an emergency exists, only one unit per patient is released at a time. Blood components other than plasma derivatives (albumin and FFP), which are stored at room temperature, must be stored only in refrigerators (or freezers) that are strictly controlled and monitored (1–6°C or 33.8–42.8°F for refrigeration). Never store any component in an unmonitored refrigerator.			
8. Recheck the physician's order.			
9. Inspect the blood component and its container for abnormalities, documenting any that are seen and notifying the transfusion service.			

Skill 36 | *(continued)*

Name _____ Date _____ Instructor _____

ACTION TAKEN	COMPLETED SUCCESSFULLY	DID NOT COMPLETE	NOTES
10. Two licensed nurses (or another qualified individual approved by the employing agency) identify the blood product and the patient. They confirm the patient's identity per #3 above. The blood product bag and tag are compared with the transfusion forms and the patient's name and bracelet identification numbers, the blood expiration date, blood group, and blood type to verify that they are the same. Document the name of anyone who verifies the patient and the component to be infused.			
11. Reassess the patient's condition and level of consciousness, ascertain vessel patency, take a full set of vital signs (temperature, pulse, respiration, and blood pressure), and document in the medical record. Abnormal vital signs require that the physician be notified, as well as documentation.			
12. Carry out proper hand hygiene. Don gloves. Initiate the transfusion at a rate of 5 ml/min or slower.			

(continues)

Skill 36 | *(continued)*

Name _____ Date _____ Instructor _____

ACTION TAKEN	COMPLETED SUCCESSFULLY	DID NOT COMPLETE	NOTES
13. Observe the patient closely, taking and recording vital signs every 5 minutes for the first 15 minutes of the transfusion. Record the time of initiation and patient's response in the record. If the patient exhibits signs or symptoms of an adverse reaction, the nurse must initiate the appropriate interventions and complete a blood transfusion reaction report.			
14. Take and record vital signs again after the infusion has been infusing for 30 minutes.			
15. Monitor and document vital signs and level of consciousness every 30 minutes until the transfusion is complete.			
16. When the transfusion is complete, flush the tubing and filter with 20–50 ml of normal saline. Take the patient's vital signs and monitor the patient's response to the transfusion.			
17. Document the time the transfusion was completed, the amount of blood infused, and the patient's response to the transfusion.			

Skill 37 | Child with Acute Diarrhea

Name _____ Date _____ Instructor _____

Approximate Time to Complete the Skill: 10–15 minutes for initial assessment with ongoing assessments based on the patient's status. Initiation of the IV will take about 15 minutes and setup of oxygen and suction equipment may take another 4–8 minutes depending on type and availability of equipment. Other tasks do not lend themselves to completion times, as they are ongoing care and safety issues.

Overview of the Skill

Accurate and timely assessment is the key to successful management and treatment of acute diarrhea in children. During the initial assessment, the nurse obtains the patient's history, elicits early recognition of signs and symptoms of dehydration and overhydration, and attempts to discover the cause of acute diarrhea. Ongoing assessment should obtain frequent vital signs, including neurological signs and hydration status, and assessing for any overall change in condition.

To determine hydration status, the nurse assesses the patient's level of consciousness, vital signs, presence and quality of pulses, capillary refill, skin condition, and presence or absence of urine output, as well as monitoring strict intake and output and monitoring laboratory values.

The patient's history will aid in diagnosing the cause of the diarrhea. Intravenous access is critical for replacement of fluids. Withholding food and fluids decreases the incidence of diarrhea and allows gastrointestinal function to return to normal. In case of an emergency, oxygen and suction are needed. A low bed and siderails keep the child safe from falls.

ACTION TAKEN	COMPLETED SUCCESSFULLY	DID NOT COMPLETE	NOTES
1. Institute systematic assessment using a head-to-toe approach, basing the assessment on clinical findings, lab values, and other monitoring systems (e.g., cardiorespiratory monitor, pulse oximeter).			
2. Maintain patency of the IV.			
3. Do not offer any food or fluids.			
4. Have oxygen and suction equipment at the bedside.			
5. Keep siderails up and the bed in low position.			